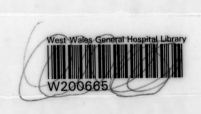

Real Whole-Body MRI

Notice

Medicine is an ever-changing science. As new research and clinical experience broaden our knowledge, changes in treatment and drug therapy are required. The authors and the publisher of this work have checked with sources believed to be reliable in their efforts to provide information that is complete and generally in accord with the standards accepted at the time of publication. However, in view of the possibility of human error or changes in medical sciences, neither the authors nor the publisher nor any other party who has been involved in the preparation or publication of this work warrants that the information contained herein is in every respect accurate or complete, and they disclaim all responsibility for any errors or omissions or for the results obtained from use of the information contained in this work. Readers are encouraged to confirm the information contained herein with other sources. For example and in particular, readers are advised to check the product information sheet included in the package of each drug they plan to administer to be certain that the information contained in this work is accurate and that changes have not been made in the recommended dose or in the contraindications for administration. This recommendation is of particular importance in connection with new or infrequently used drugs.

Real Whole-Body MRI
Requirements, Indications, Perspectives

Edited by

Mathias Goyen, MD
University Medical Center Hamburg-Eppendorf
Hamburg, Germany

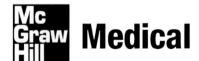

New York • Chicago • San Francisco • Lisbon • London • Madrid • Mexico City
New Delhi • San Juan • Seoul • Singapore • Sydney • Toronto

Real Whole-Body MRI: Requirements, Indications, Perspectives

1 2 3 4 5 6 7 8 9 0 CTP/CTP 0 9 8 7

ISBN 978-0-07-149867-8
MHID 0-07-149867-2

This book was set by Type-Design, Berlin.
The editor was Ruth Weinberg.
The production supervisor was Phil Galea.
The English translation was by mt-g medical translation, Ulm.
The cover designer was Mary McKeon. Photo credits: *Left:* Medical scans
(Digital Composite) RF. Don Farrall/Getty Images; *Right:* Spinal cord. RM.
@Firefly Productions/CORBIS.
China Translation & Printing Service, Ltd., was printer and binder.

This book is printed on acid-free paper.

Previously published in 2006 by ABW Wissenschaftsverlag GmbH, Berlin,
Germany.

Library of Congress Cataloging-in-Publication Data

Real whole body MRI : requirements, indications, perspectives / Mathias Goyen, ed.
    p. ; cm.
  Includes bibliographical references and index.
  ISBN-13: 978-0-07-149867-8 (alk. paper)
  ISBN-10: 0-07-149867-2 (alk. paper)
 1. Magnetic resonance imaging--Diagnostic use. 2. Whole body imaging. I.
Goyen, Mathias.
  [DNLM: 1. Whole Body Imaging. 2. Magnetic Resonance Imaging. WN 185 R288
2008] RC78.7.N83R43 2008 616.07'548--dc22
                    2007020149

Table of contents

Technology

Clinical applications

Preface

The introduction of high-resolution whole-body magnetic resonance imaging is based on the rapid and intensive advancement of various magnetic resonance tomographic examination techniques, as well as new methods in data processing. The editor and authors have made crucial contributions towards establishing whole-body MRI in various investigative settings, rendering it more precise and applying it for diverse indications. The work presented here is founded upon the extensive experience of the editor, as well as drawing upon the broad range of experience from other scientific working groups. The first section of the book is dedicated to the technical requirements of whole-body MRI, as well as the principles and the associated data processing, whereas all aspects of whole-body MRI are presented from a clinical perspective in the subsequent chapters. This includes examination techniques, an update of the clinical questions posed, and a richly illustrated presentation of the clinical areas of cardiovascular investigation and musculoskeletal diseases. Oncological whole-body imaging tackles the comparison of whole-body MRI with bone scintigraphy in the detection of bone metastases, and with FDG-PET in respect to whole-body tumor staging. Both the clinical and experimental questions concerning whole-body MRI are addressed in detail.

The book represents a crucial contribution towards the rapid propagation and clinical integration of whole-body MRI. This book is outstanding by virtue of its clear structure, the excellent image examples and also the clinical concept.

I wish this book all the success it deserves!

Prof. Dr. med. Thomas Vogl

Foreword

In modern MRI, the advent of movable surface coils, ultra-fast gradient technology and multi-channel receivers (≥ 8 channels) have propelled whole-body MRI from conception to implementation. The latest 32 channel systems allow simultaneous imaging from numerous receiver coil matrices. This, coupled with automated table movement and image fusion and montage postprocessing software, make whole-body MRI not only feasible but also practical. Whole-body MR imaging times have decreased drastically from over an hour to perform one pulse sequence on the whole body to less than an hour to perform multiple pulse sequences on the whole body for a comprehensive examination. Whole-body MR imaging and angiography advances have thus begat a whole family of clinical whole-body MR applications.

The key to exploring new technology is separating the clinically relevant applications from the simple academic curiosity of scientists which may be costly and clinically irrelevant or worse yet, potentially harmful. In an age where CT has become today's plain film equivalent, I sometimes think medical clinicians have forgotten that X-rays are potentially harmful. After all, Europeans have kept better sight of the fact that indiscriminate use of X-rays could have serious negative impact on the general population and thus many European countries regulate the use CT. Following suit, the United States Food and Drug Administration has recently labeled X-rays a carcinogen. Thus MRI is poised to become a very powerful whole-body screening tool because it lacks the two major pitfalls that plagued whole-body CT, namely ionizing radiation and iodinated contrast material. Whole-body MRI has great potential advantage over the competing modalities of PET and CT for not only early detection of primary disease but also surveillance for local and metastatic spread of tumor. Oncogenic osteomalacia and other more systemic syndromes may also be facilely evaluated by whole-body MR, but proof of these concepts lies ahead.

My esteemed colleague and friend Dr. Mathias Goyen has been working extensively in the field of MRI over the last years and has made seminal contributions toward expanding the scope of whole-body MR applications and making it clinically practical and effective. This book, to my knowledge, is the first of its kind and offers a hands-on approach to the evolving field of whole-body MRI, which gives the reader the tools to effectively utilize and optimize application of whole-body MRI technology in the patient care setting.

F. Scott Pereles, MD
Salinas Valley Radiologists
559 Abbott St
Salinas, CA 93901

Salinas, Summer 2006

Foreword and acknowledgements

Technical advances in medical technology today allow the performance of high-resolution whole-body magnetic resonance imaging (MRI) examinations of the body from an onco-logical perspective in a single examination. Whole-body MRI, as a young, future-shaping imaging technique, has therefore fundamentally changed the direction of discussions on the use of MR technology in oncological secondary prevention. Although whole-body MRI is just in the early stages of its development, the enormous medical and economic poten-tial is already plain to see. The aim of this book is to provide a current overview of this new and multifaceted field of modern MRI radiology. Following introductory chapters on technology, the majority of the book is dedicated to clinical fields of application for whole-body MRI. I would like to thank all authors for their valuable contribution and dedicated collaboration, which made this current compilation of essential aspects of whole-body MRI possible. Thank you to my publisher, Dr. Axel Bedürftig, for his uncomplicated, construc-tive and always friendly collaboration and for his strong efforts to make an English edition of the book possible. Special thanks go to my radiology teacher and mentor, Jörg F. Deba-tin, MD, MBA, Medical Director and CEO of the University Medical Center Hamburg-Ep-pendorf, who followed and very much supported this book project.

Mathias Goyen   Hamburg, July 2006

Author index

Gerald Antoch, MD
Assistant Professor of Radiology
Department of Diagnostic and Interventional Radiology and Neuroradiology
University Hospital Essen
Hufelandstrasse 55
45147 Essen
Germany
e-mail: gerald.antoch@uni-essen.de

Andreas Bockisch, MD, PhD
Chairman
Department of Nuclear Medicine
University Hospital Essen
Hufelandstrasse 55
45147 Essen
Germany
e-mail: andreas.bockisch@uni-essen.de

Nadir Ghanem, MD
Department of Diagnostic Radiology
University Hospital Freiburg
Hugstetter Strasse 55
79106 Freiburg
Germany
e-mail: gha@mrs1.ukl.uni-freiburg.de

Mathias Goyen, MD
University Medical Center Hamburg-Eppendorf
Martinistrasse 52
20246 Hamburg
Germany
e-mail: goyen@uke.uni-hamburg.de

Joachim Graessner, MS
Siemens AG
Medical Solutions
Region Hanse, ES BMG MR
Koenigsreihe 22
22041 Hamburg
Germany
e-mail: joachim.graessner@siemens.com

Christoph U. Herborn, MD
Medical Prevention Center Hamburg (MPCH)
University Medical Center Hamburg-Eppendorf
Falkenried 88
20251 Hamburg
Germany
e-mail: herborn@mpch.de

Alexander Huppertz, MD
Imaging Science Institute Charité – Siemens
Robert-Koch-Platz 7
10115 Berlin
Germany
e-mail: alexander.huppertz@siemens.com

Mark E. Ladd, PhD
Professor and Director of Biomedical Imaging
Department of Diagnostic and Interventional Radiology and Neuroradiology
University Hospital Essen
Hufelandstrasse 55
45147 Essen
Germany
e-mail: mark.ladd@uni-essen.de

Susanne C. Ladd, MD, MS
Associate Professor of Radiology
Department of Diagnostic and Interventional Radiology and Neuroradiology
University Hospital Essen
Hufelandstrasse 55
45147 Essen
Germany
e-mail: susanne.ladd@uni-duisburg-essen.de

Thomas C. Lauenstein, MD
Assistant Professor of Radiology
The Emory Clinic
1365 Clifton Road, Bldg A, Suite AT-627
Atlanta, GA 30322
USA
e-mail: tlauens@emory.edu

Sabine Lenk, MD
Department of Diagnostic Radiology
Eberhard-Karls-University Tubingen,
Hoppe-Seyler-Strasse 3
72076 Tübingen
Germany
e-mail: sabine.lenk@mri-online.de

Konstantin Nikolaou, MD
Department of Clinical Radiology
Ludwig-Maximilians-University Munich
Großhadern Campus
Marchioninistrasse 15
81377 München
Germany
konstantin.nikolaou@med.uni-muenchen.de

Harald H. Quick, PhD
Associate Professor of Biomedical Imaging
Department of Diagnostic and Interventional Radiology and Neuroradiology
University Hospital Essen
Hufelandstrasse 55
45147 Essen
Germany
e-mail: hhquick@uni-essen.de

Heinz-Peter Schlemmer, MD, MS
Department of Diagnostic Radiology
Eberhard-Karls-University Tubingen,
Hoppe-Seyler-Strasse 3
72076 Tübingen
Germany
e-mail: heinz-peter.schlemmer@med.uni-tuebingen.de

Michael Thali, MD
Institute of Forensic Medicine
University of Bern
Bühlstrasse 20
3012 Bern
Switzerland
e-mail: michael.thali@irm.unibe.ch

Patrick Veit-Haibach, MD
Department of Nuclear Medicine
University Hospital Zurich
Rämistrasse 100
8091 Zürich
Switzerland
e-mail: patrick.veit-haibach@usz.ch

Florian M. Vogt, MD
Assistant Professor of Radiology
Department of Diagnostic and Interventional Radiology and Neuroradiology
University Hospital Essen
Hufelandstrasse 55
45147 Essen
Germany
e-mail: florian.vogt@uni-essen.de

Introduction: Whole-body imaging – Diagnostic strategy of the future?

Mathias Goyen

Since the discovery of X-rays more than 110 years ago, radiology has made tremendous progress. Especially in the last 30 years, the decisive breakthrough has been achieved with the introduction of the cross-sectional imaging techniques computed tomography (CT) and magnetic resonance imaging (MRI), as well as important advancements in the field of interventional radiology and nuclear medicine.

Radiological imaging has become very accurate over the years, with high sensitivities and specificities compared with the respective standard of reference; data can be acquired three-dimensionally and presented to clinicians.

Functional imaging has become reality, and it is expected that molecular imaging will also find its way into clinical use. New, organ-specific contrast agents for all imaging modalities, in particular for MRI, are undergoing clinical testing. With the help of new imaging strategies, patients can be examined quickly; this means that even examinations with expensive machines are economically viable, as a high patient throughput leads to reduced costs.

The aforementioned progress of the last 30 years has become possible thanks to developments in the fields of information technology and computer science. The performance of computers has doubled every 18 months over the last 15 years (Moore's Law). Computers and medical devices have become smaller in size, and image acquisition, resolution and image transmission have appreciably improved and have contributed to further progress in medical imaging over the last 20 years.

These developments have especially influenced the cross-sectional techniques CT and MRI, both for which fast data acquisition has brought about a significant increase in patient throughput.

For cost reasons, these cross-sectional techniques were for a long period only deployed in stepwise diagnostics once the conventional X-ray images or ultrasound had already been obtained. As a result of the reduction in acquisition times for CT and MRI, the additional costs in comparison with conventional X-ray technology have fallen. These higher costs are clearly put into perspective when the additional information derived through the use of cross-sectional imaging techniques is taken into consideration. CT examinations of the lung have already replaced conventional X-ray recordings for many applications; there has also been a significant worldwide reduction in the number of barium X-ray diagnostic examinations of the abdomen or in urology for example; here, CT is now often the examination mode of choice.

Regional – Global

The same technical advances, which through faster data acquisition lead to a reduction in examination costs, lead to a paradigm shift in cross-sectional imaging away from focused examination towards whole-body imaging. Until a few years ago this was not possible, i.e. radiological imaging was limited to the depiction of a single region of the body for each examination.

There were several reasons for this limitation: Above all were the aforementioned absence of technical options as well as limitations placed by contrast agents and reasons of radiation protection.

Whole-body CT

For several years now, so-called multi-slice CT systems, which allow whole-body examinations, have been available in clinical routine work. An important consideration with whole-body CT is the significant radiation exposure which sometimes arises. In the case of a seriously injured patient with compelling reasons for the diagnosis to be performed promptly, this radiation exposure is certainly justified, as it is with intensive care patients e.g. with the indication of a focus search for sepsis.

The use of CT for the early detection of diseases (prevention), on the other hand, is rightly subject to controversial discussion – especially in Europe. In recent years, vehicle fleets with mobile CT systems are out and about in the US offering their services. The health conscious in the US can nowadays even be examined with whole-body CT in shopping malls.

The Food and Drug Administration (FDA) still has no data to document the benefit of a whole-body CT examination. Large American specialist associations (American College of Radiology, American College of Cardiology, American Heart Association) therefore do not recommend whole-body CT examinations for screening purposes.

Whole-body MRI

Just as the technical advancement in the field of CT made whole-body imaging possible, today we are in a position to image the entire body with a single MRI examination (Chaps. 1 and 2). This is largely attributable to the enormous technical progress in the field of MRI gradient technology over recent years, as well as the development of organ-specific contrast agents (Chap. 9). Another factor is the development of rolling table platforms (e.g. AngioSURF), which allow the patient to be moved through the magnetic tunnel. Advantages of MRI compared with CT examination firstly include the absence of radiation exposure, and secondly the fact that MR contrast agents show an excellent safety profile and can be used e.g. for patients with kidney insufficiency or hyperthyroidism.

Various indications for whole-body MRI – both oncological and non-oncological – have already been clinically evaluated. For instance, whole-body MRI can be deployed for patients with bone metastases as an alternative to the standard of reference, bone scintigraphy (Chaps. 6 and 7) or in comparison with FDG-PET (Chap. 8). In contrast to scintigraphy, in which tumor-induced activity in osteoblasts is a prerequisite, in MRI the large number of protons in the tumor matrix allows direct detection. Compared with scintigraphy, an MRI examination allows assessment of soft tissue and parenchymal organs at the same time as bone metastases, and an overview of the patient's overall tumor load can be obtained.

Additional potential indications are whole-body fat measurement by means of MRI to determine body composition (Chap. 10) and the imaging of muscular infections in patients with polymyositis (Chap. 5). Whole-body MR angiography has already made advances in routine diagnostics, on account of atherosclerosis being a widespread disease thus requiring extensive diagnostic attention (Chap. 3).

A further indication for whole-body MRI is autopsy of the deceased. Initial studies from Switzerland (Chap. 13) indicate that MRI can be a useful supplement for autopsy, especially for patients for whom a conventional autopsy is not possible due to the absence of consent by the relatives on religious grounds.

Early detection of diseases

Today's patient goes to the doctor even in good health so as not to become sick in the first place. The trend is prevention. Prevention has many aspects; the most important ones are cardiovascular risk factors, which have risen to shocking proportions since the Second World War and have now become widespread diseases. Experiences with radiological screening techniques are limited. The most noteworthy are X-ray thorax screening examinations for tuberculosis in Europe in the 1960s and 1970s and mammography screening in the 1980s and 1990s.

The advantages of the MRI technique (latest hardware developments, absence of side effects and high diagnostic accuracy) make MRI appear to be especially well suited for the early detection of diseases (Chaps. 11 and 12).

As the costs for a whole-body MRI examination are still too high to allow this technique to be used in individualized screening examinations, a solution possibly lies in the combination of several MR-based separate examinations to form a comprehensive MR screening protocol. The image quality attained in this examination is comparable with the image quality that can be achieved for each separate examination. Of course, no conclusions can be drawn from the current data status as to the general value of MRI screening, as a far greater number of cases is required. Moreover, screening can only be medically appropriate given a concise definition of the risk groups. It is obvious that a screening examination may be advantageous for the individual if e.g. a kidney or liver cell carcinoma, which is not symptomatic, is discovered. Future studies must e.g. compare the costs for this screening with the life-years saved.

It is essential when deploying imaging techniques for screening purposes, especially MRI, that the radiologists working in preventative medicine are careful about what they see on the images. They have to be aware of the limitations of the methods, the variations and signs of wear of the human body, and provide an appropriate assessment during the medical consultation with the customer to avoid the customer being a victim of the so-called "VOMIT" syndrome (victim of modern imaging technology).

Whole-body diagnostics for prevention purposes should, under all circumstances, be integrated into a comprehensive prevention and screening concept, which, besides a clinical examination, should ideally include a survey of laboratory parameters and functional examinations, such as ergometry, as well as lifestyle coaching based on the results obtained.

Summary

- Cross-sectional imaging techniques have replaced conventional X-ray examinations as the examination mode of choice.
- Whole-body examinations have become feasible as a result of the enormous progress in the field of medical technology and advancements in contrast agent research. There are essentially two modalities available: CT and MRI.
- Whole-body CT examination is mainly used for severely injured and intensive care patients.
- Whole-body MRI examination has already been successfully used in various oncological and non-oncological investigations. Screening for diseases may represent a new indication for whole-body MRI. In contrast to CT, MRI is not accompanied by radiation exposure. Whole-body diagnostics should definitely be just one part of a comprehensive prevention and early detection concept.

Technology

1 Technical requirements for whole-body MRI

Harald H. Quick, Mark E. Ladd

1.1 Introduction

MRI examinations are traditionally limited to areas, which can be covered by the MR field of view (FOV). These are typically less than 50 cm. Certain investigations however require a larger volume of the patient to be covered, e.g. examinations of the spinal column, MR angiography (MRA) examinations of the pelvis-leg region or whole-body MRI metastasis search. Strategies for enlarging the effective MRI image area must be developed for these examinations. Multistation techniques, with which adjacent individual, slightly overlapping stations are acquired, have therefore been developed to effectively expand the FOV. There is also a trend towards ever shorter magnet designs that also further reduce the useable FOV (< 40 cm). A shorter magnet generally improves acceptance among claustrophobic and overweight patients. A smaller FOV also tends to reduce the risk of nerve stimulation because of the shortened gradient system, which allows shorter gradient switching times (higher slew rates) and therefore faster imaging. However, to exploit these inherent advantages of shorter magnets with an effectively larger FOV – up to and including whole-body applications – the relevant technical requirements must be met.

1.2 Hardware

Generally, the useable FOV of an MR scanner is essentially defined by three hardware groups and their related parameters: 1. The main magnet with its homogeneity over the imaging volume; 2. The gradient system with its linearity over the imaging volume; and 3. The radiofrequency (RF) system with its RF signal homogeneity and signal sensitivity over the imaging volume. Whole-body MRI imposes very special demands on these system components of the scanner hardware.

1.2.1 Main magnet

The magnet of a whole-body MR scanner should have a high main magnetic field strength to provide sufficient equilibrium magnetization and therefore a high potential signal-to-noise ratio (SNR) for good image quality. MRI at field strengths above 1.0 Tesla – or better yet 1.5 Tesla (Fig. 1.1) – is currently viewed as the standard and is increasingly being supplemented with 3 Tesla systems in clinical use. The homogeneity of the basic magnetic field over the examination volume should be as high as possible to ensure low image distortion and high signal homogeneity. The homogeneous examination volume should be as large as possible to capture the full extent of the patient's body without artifacts (Fig. 1.2) and distortions. A cylindrical design of the main magnet is conformant with all these requirements and therefore currently represents the most frequently occurring magnet design (Fig. 1.1).

2

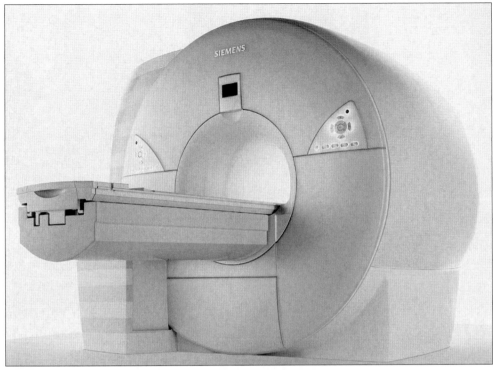

Figure 1.1 Modern 1.5 Tesla whole-body MR scanner with cylindrical design ("Avanto", Siemens Medical Solutions, Erlangen, Germany). The dimensions of the magnet aperture represent the current norm of approximately 160 cm length with a 60 cm diameter (Photo: Siemens).

1.2.2 Gradients

Special demands are also placed on the gradient system in order to be able to realize whole-body MR examinations: A fast gradient slew rate combined with a high gradient amplitude are the prerequisites for short repetition and echo times (TR and TE) and thus for fast imaging and coverage of a large examination volume in the shortest possible time. This can be seen as a fundamental prerequisite for clinically acceptable examination times for the large volumes of whole-body MRI. A high degree of gradient linearity over a large area is required to keep image distortion in and around the imaging FOV to a minimum (Fig. 1.3). These requirements can also be best realized with a cylindrical design of the gradient system.

1.2.3 RF system

A radiofrequency system suitable for whole-body MRI is characterized by RF excitation with a homogeneous signal excitation over as large an examination volume as possible. Here it is important that the excitation flip angle remains as constant as feasible, as the image contrast is fundamentally influenced by this parameter. Large cylindrical volume coils,

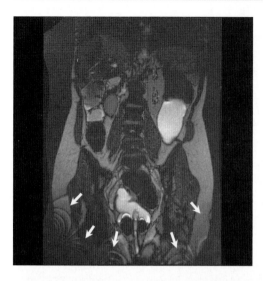

Figure 1.2 Magnetic field homogeneity. Coronal MR image with a large FOV (50 cm) to demonstrate the effect of the magnetic field homogeneity of the main magnet. In this TrueFISP sequence, which is very sensitive to homogeneity, there are black ring artifacts shown on the margins of the FOV (arrows) – a consequence of signal obliteration in the inhomogeneous region of the magnet.

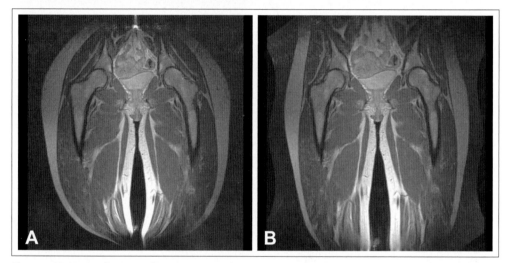

Figure 1.3A, B Gradient non-linearity. Coronal MR images with a large FOV (50 cm) without **(A)** and with **(B)** distortion correction of gradient non-linearities. Without distortion correction **(A)**, the images with a large FOV show structures with significant distortion on the margins. To a certain extent these distortions can be compensated for with image processing **(B)**, such that the individual stations or FOVs can be combined to form a single large image FOV for use in whole-body MRI.

like the RF whole-body coils fitted inside the magnet tunnel, are used here as they fulfill this requirement.

In terms of signal reception, homogeneous RF signal reception over as large an examination region as possible is on the list of requirements; however, homogeneity plays a lesser role here compared with signal sensitivity, as inhomogeneous reception intensity only affects the brightness distribution over the volume, but not the underlying image contrast. In regard to the homogeneous volume, the whole-body RF coil also offers an ad-

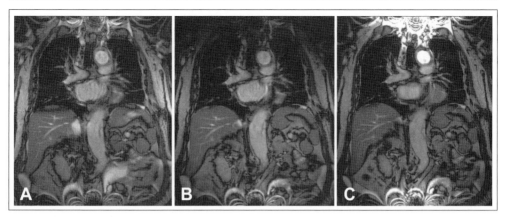

Figure 1.4A–C Radiofrequency signal homogeneity. Coronal MR image with large FOV (50 cm) acquired **(A)** with the built-in whole-body RF coil of the scanner. The image in **(A)** appears noisy, with a low SNR and therefore poor image quality, but it nevertheless demonstrates a high level of signal homogeneity. In comparison, the use of RF surface coils in **(B)** delivers a higher SNR and therefore improved image quality. The signal is however locally restricted to the individual coil elements located in the lower half of the image, which severely limits the illumination and signal homogeneity at the upper edge of the image and forces RF coil elements to be placed over the entire FOV for complete coverage of the anatomical region **(C)**.

vantage here. For signal reception and the maximum SNR attainable with such a large volume coil, a coil of this type is however extremely limited. Hence, diverse concepts with RF surface coils have come into use. Surface coils are placed directly over the examination region and receive signals from the immediate vicinity of the examination volume. At the same time, these coils detect the unavoidable noise from a relatively limited region, so that the potential SNR attainable with these coils is relatively high. At the same time, the disadvantage of surface coils lies in their severely restricted sensitivity range. Several coil elements of this type are required to cover larger anatomical regions (Fig. 1.4); they can be combined together as phased-array surface coils. Phased-array coils allow optimization of the SNR while extending the region for signal reception. A prerequisite for exploiting the advantages inherent in this type of coil technology is a large number of RF receivers to which the coil elements can be connected either individually or in groups. This is also a basic prerequisite for the use of parallel imaging acquisition techniques.

1.3 Multistation techniques

One possibility of extending the effective FOV is to divide the examination into several discrete partial examinations, whereby the patient table together with the patient is moved relative to the imaging volume in-between the partial measurements [1–4]. With these so-called multistation techniques, the fact is exploited that different body regions lie sequentially in the imaging region defined and limited by magnet homogeneity, gradient linearity, and RF signal excitation and reception. The previously defined list of conventional limitations remains applicable for each partial imaging field with this method; however, in this way the effective FOV may be expanded over several stations.

The basic requirement for the implementation of multistation techniques is the technical capability to move the patient table relative to the imaging field of the MR scanner. Here the maximum range of movement of the table directly determines the effective FOV, which can be covered stepwise with an examination of this type. Older generation MR systems typically have a range of movement limited to less than 150 cm. To examine a patient from head to toe it is therefore unavoidable to reposition the patient at least once during the examination. For example, in the first phase the patient is positioned head-first, in the second phase feet-first.

For signal reception the multistation techniques initially used the whole-body RF coil, which however only provided a moderate SNR and consequently limited image quality. Later, various concepts were introduced using RF surface coils, with the aim to significantly raise the attainable image quality through higher SNR.

1.3.1 Peripheral coils

MR angiography (MRA) of the pelvis-leg region may be viewed as the driving clinical application for the development of table movement techniques. The limitations of a conventional FOV were overcome for the first time through the expansion of this anatomical region to an examination region of 120–140 cm. After initial attempts with the RF whole-body coil of the scanner [1–3, 8], which were limited by signal reception, solutions with motorized table movement combined with RF surface coils were increasingly applied [4, 9, 10].

The useable range of movement and therefore the effective FOV of these initial table movement techniques was around 150 cm, which corresponds to three or four stations, a distance sufficient for peripheral vessel studies. The various peripheral RF surface coils (Fig. 1.5) specially developed for this application also covered the target examination region, either on their own or in combination with additional RF coils.

The technical requirements for a stationwise expansion of the effective FOV with a high SNR and concomitant high image quality were thus established. Nevertheless, clinical needs and requirements were soon aimed towards further expansion of the FOV to possible whole-body MR applications [11].

1.3.2 Moving table platforms: SKIP, Angio*SURF* etc.

To overcome the limited range of movement of the patient table and to avoid having to reposition the patient during whole-body MRI, crucial impetus was provided by independent research groups for technical implementations to achieve "real" whole-body MRI. Manually movable table platforms were developed, e.g. "SKIP" (Stepping Kinematic Imaging Platform, Magnetic Moments, Bloomfield, MI, USA) [12] and "Angio*SURF*" (Angiographic System for Unlimited Rolling Field-of-views, MR-Innovation GmbH, Essen, Germany) [13–15], which exceeded the range of movement of the motorized patient tables used in MR scanners, thereby extending the achievable FOV to approx. 200 cm and giving rise to "real" whole-body MRI. Stepwise whole-body MRI now became possible with five to six stations.

The inadequate coverage of this examination field with RF surface coils was circumvented with the elegant solution of an RF surface coil pair positioned stationary in the

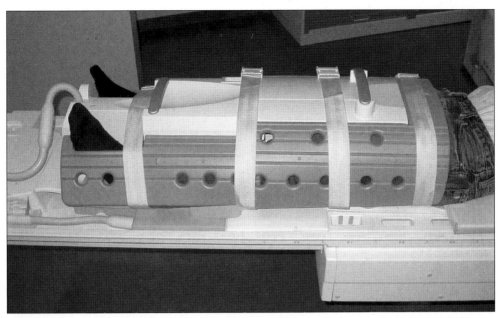

Figure 1.5 Dedicated peripheral "phased-array" RF surface coil (Siemens Medical Solutions, Erlangen, Germany) for the acquisition of multistation MR angiography (MRA) examinations of the pelvis-leg vasculature. The phased-array coil provides expanded anatomical coverage, as well as a high local SNR for enhanced image quality.

isocenter of the magnet (Fig. 1.6) A phased-array coil is integrated into the patient table for this purpose, which delivers signals from the posterior region of the patient. On the anterior of the patient, mounted on a coil glider, is a second phased array surface coil, which is height-adjustable and held in position by two arms at the isocenter of the magnet, thereby allowing the coil glider to adapt to the contour of the patient passing through the magnet tunnel. The patient is positioned on an MR-compatible table platform mounted on rollers.

Using this technique, the patient can be quickly pulled stepwise through the magnet passing between the two surface coils (Fig. 1.6). The RF surface coils provide the SNR required for high image quality without having to completely enclose the patient in RF coils from head to toe. The technique has been applied extensively in clinical use in whole-body MRA [12–17] (Fig. 1.7A), whole-body metastasis screening of oncological patients [18–21] (Fig. 1.7B), and as part of MR-based preventive examinations [22, 23]. The phased-array RF surface coils used here facilitate the use of parallel acquisition techniques to enhance spatial resolution [15].

1.3.3   Matrix coils – Coil elements from head to toe

The latest generation of MR scanners increasingly offers integration of these requirements for whole-body MRI: a table movement range of over 200 cm, integrated concepts for covering the patient's body with a large number of dedicated phased-array RF surface coils, as well as a large number of RF receivers for signal management of these coil elements.

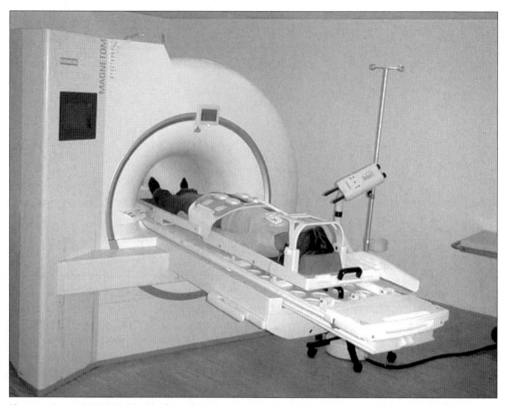

Figure 1.6 Angio*SURF* table platform (MR-Innovation GmbH, Essen, Germany) mounted on the examination table of a Siemens Sonata MR scanner with a patient lying on top. The table and coil position are shown for the third of five stations; for purposes of illustration, the table has been moved outside of the magnet: for the actual measurement the coil glider is positioned in the iso-center. For the MR whole-body examination, five contiguous 3D data sets are acquired from head to toe. The patient is moved manually on the platform between each data set. As the table is moved, the patient slides between a fixed RF receiver coil located posteriorly and a receiver coil mounted anteriorly on the coil glider. The glider follows the contour of the patient, which minimizes the separation of the coil to the patient, thereby optimizing the signal-to-noise ratio and the image quality. An additional frame protects the patient's face. The technique allows a fast MRI whole-body examination with high image quality (see Fig. 1.7).

The aim is to cover the patient from head to toe with a uniform distribution of highly sensitive surface coils to ensure the best possible signal sensitivity from the entire body. Siemens (Siemens Medical Solutions, Erlangen, Germany) offers an RF system of this type with up to 76 coil elements (newest systems with up to 102 coil elements) and up to 32 receiver channels with a 205 cm table movement range under the name "Tim" (Total Imaging Matrix) (Fig. 1.8). Through the use of dedicated surface coils adapted to the respective examination region and through the large number of RF receivers, this system fully exploits the potentially achievable SNR. The individual coil elements can be flexibly combined with the available receiver channels. As with the techniques previously cited, here the state-of-the-art is the stepwise motorized movement of the patient and the associated data acquisition in discrete stations.

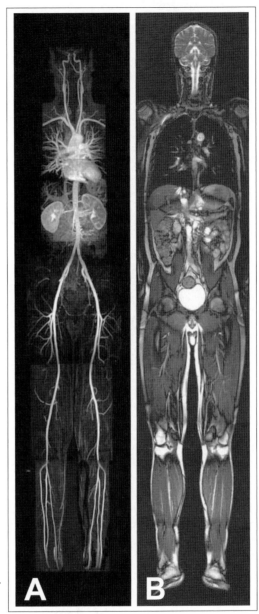

Figure 1.7A, B Whole-body MR angiography **(A)** combined from five individual 3D data sets, which were acquired over a total period of 72 seconds. Contrast agent was injected during image acquisition. Besides MR angiography, the Angio*SURF* system can also be deployed as a staging method for metastasis search in patients with metastatic disease (Body*SURF*) **(B)**. Here the examination protocol encompasses MR imaging of the soft tissue and the bones.

1.3.4 Software

With the emergence of multistation MR techniques, not only were hardware developments required, such as dedicated RF coil concepts and table movement, but software requirements also changed in parallel: 1. RF coils need to be switchable between the stations so that only the coils in the respective imaging volume actively contribute to signal acquisition. 2. The prescan to determine the adjustment parameters, such as tuning, shimming,

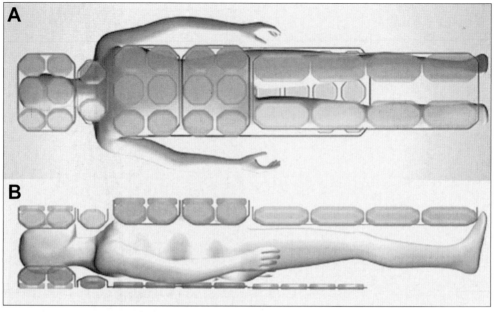

Figure 1.8A, B Schematic representation of "Tim" (Total imaging matrix) RF technology (Siemens Medical Solutions, Erlangen, Germany) in a top view **(A)** and side view **(B)**. The patient can be covered with a full complement of dedicated RF surface coils. Up to 76 coil elements can be linked with up to 32 independent RF receivers in various modes to form an RF matrix. The whole-body coverage of the patient with separate RF surface coils in combination with motorized table movement permits whole-body image acquisition with a relatively high SNR and, furthermore, the combination with parallel imaging techniques (Photo: Siemens).

specific absorption rate (SAR), excitation flip angle, etc. needs to be carried out and stored for each station separate from the actual examination, so that these time-consuming parameters can be determined for all stations prior to a potentially time-critical application such as contrast-enhanced MRA. 3. The section stacks for data acquisition at each station need to be individually positioned and angulated and variable in their respective local resolution (matrix, section thickness), thereby allowing individual adaptation to the anatomical situation of each station.

1.3.5 Parallel imaging

The use of phased-array RF surface coils along with the availability of RF receiver channels for the multistation techniques forms the basis for the application of parallel imaging techniques to whole-body MRI. Parallel imaging itself takes on a special role in whole-body MRI. Besides the acknowledged advantages of parallel imaging, e.g. artifact reduction in examinations of the thoracic-abdominal region through shorter breath holding, the total time savings is multiplied by the number of stations required to cover the body volume. Parallel imaging allows larger anatomical regions to be captured per unit time or the local resolution to be raised in the same acquisition time (assuming a sufficient SNR) or a combination of both effects. This is an important consideration, especially in whole-body MRI, for capturing the larger anatomical regions within a clinically acceptable time with an adequate spatial resolution.

By using parallel imaging techniques, on the other hand, the already large quantities of data involved in whole-body MRI are further expanded through the use of matrix coils, through numerous receiver channels, and through the acquisition of large volumes over several stations while maintaining a high spatial resolution. The demands placed on image reconstruction, database management, archiving media, etc. are enormous and therefore present further development potential and requirements.

1.4   Something is moving: Move during scan – Continuous table movement

The multistation MR techniques previously described still possess some potential disadvantages: The time taken for table movement is not available for data acquisition, and the table movement between stations typically lasts between three and four seconds; the partial FOVs for each station typically overlap slightly, requiring additional time for redundant data acquisition; time is necessary at each station for the reestablishment of the steady state; signal attenuation often arises on the margins of the FOVs which can lead to inhomogeneities in the resulting combined overview images; and non-linearities in the gradient system lead to geometric distortions on the margins of the partial FOVs, which in turn can cause artifacts on the boundaries between adjacent stations. Many of these disadvantages hamper the evaluation of the images, especially on the boundaries of the partial FOVs. The ideal situation would be a continuous data set with uninterrupted and unchanging quality, which can be processed as a whole during image viewing and assessment.

Various techniques for data acquisition during continuous table movement have been investigated as alternatives to the multistation techniques. In the simplest methods, fast two-dimensional (2D) axially oriented sections are acquired in the isocenter of the magnet during continuous table movement and are subsequently combined [24, 25]. If the table speed is so slow that the table movement is less than the acquired section thickness, the image artifacts are then tolerable.

Fast 2D axial section acquisition with continuous table movement is subject to some restrictions: Limited in-plane resolution and relatively large section thicknesses restrict the possibility of reconstructing the axially acquired data in the coronal or sagittal planes; in addition, until now only a small number of image contrasts (gradient echo or EPI variants) have been made available. The conventional multistation techniques, on the other hand, offer high spatial resolution and the complete range of MR image contrasts, whereby they suffer from the limitations stated above – the temporal ineffectiveness and possible artifacts at the margins of the partial FOVs. Ideally, a combination of the advantages of both methods should be sought.

Methods recently developed pursue just this strategy. They allow either phase encoding [26] or frequency encoding [27–31] along the movement axis during table movement, which facilitates 2D and 3D data acquisition. These techniques for continuous table movement during data acquisition, also termed "Move During Scan (MDS)" techniques, place special requirements on data acquisition, hardware and image reconstruction: Inhomogeneity of the main magnetic field (Fig. 1.2) and non-linearity of the gradients (Fig. 1.3) generate image distortions at the margins of the FOV, which are now a function of time, because

11

the table is moved through the tomograph during acquisition [32]. In addition, a number of adjustment parameters, which previously were modified once per station for the station-wise examination of the patient, must now be automatically adapted during table movement. These parameters include the tuning of the RF transmit coil, the transmit and receive frequency, the RF transmission power, the RF receiver gain, the "shimming" of the magnet, the activation of the RF surface coil elements located in the imaging region and other parameters, all of which are needed to ensure optimal, homogeneous image quality and the safety of the patient. Otherwise, the excitation flip angle can, for instance, have a different value in the pelvic region than in the thoracic region and the image contrast varies unpredictably. Even without a complete solution for adapting these parameters "on the fly", initial studies with MDS techniques show promising results with volunteers [33, 34] and patients [34, 35] (Fig. 1.9). Parallel imaging techniques can also be applied here through the use of surface coils combined with independent RF receivers [34, 36], and the potential for faster imaging, larger anatomical coverage in the same time, and/or improved spatial resolution can be exploited.

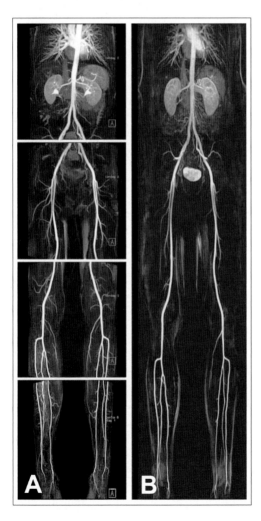

Figure 1.9A, B Contrast-enhanced peripheral MRA **(A)** compared with the "Move During Scan" (MDS) technique **(B)**, with which continuous data acquisition takes place during patient table movement. The multistation technique requires acquisition of several discrete, slightly overlapping FOVs (A), whereas the MDS technique delivers a large, seamless FOV. With the multistation technique gradient distortions – as shown in Fig. 1.3 – on the edges of the individual FOVs potentially lead to discontinuity artifacts.

Both technologies have the potential to be expanded to whole-body MRI from head to toe (courtesy: Michael O. Zenge, MS, University Hospital Essen, Germany).

The application of such MDS techniques is potentially rewarded with the depiction of extended anatomical structures in large seamless images and has the potential of achieving a paradigm shift in MR data acquisition, reconstruction, postprocessing and evaluation.

1.5 Short magnet systems: How much magnet does whole-body MRI need?

In terms of magnet design, an unabated trend towards ever-shorter magnets with as large of FOV as possible continues. The state-of-the-art for cylindrical 1.5 Tesla tomographs can be considered a magnet length of approx. 140–160 cm coupled with a homogeneous volume of 40–50 cm length. With the multistation techniques, the number of stations required to achieve whole-body coverage of the patient is directly dependent on the length of the useable homogeneous FOV. A short useable FOV therefore necessitates the acquisition and sequencing of many individual stations. MR systems with short cylindrical magnets, such as the "Espree" from Siemens, present another special challenge for whole-body MRI in this regard.

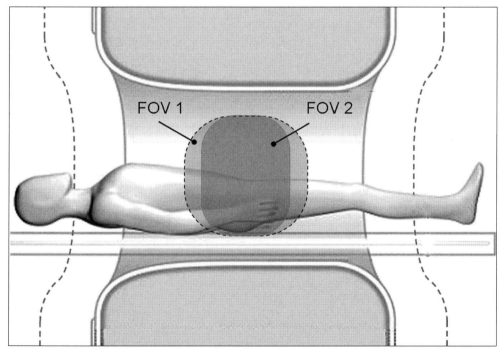

Figure 1.10 Schematic representation of a longitudinal section through a cylindrical short magnet ("Espree", Siemens Medical Solutions, Erlangen, Germany). Whereas conventional 1.5 Tesla magnets have a bore length of typically approx. 160 cm (dashed line) and a bore diameter of typically approx. 60 cm, this short magnet with the same field strength has a magnet length of just approximately 125 cm with a wider bore diameter of approximately 70 cm. Compared to the homogeneous FOV of a standard magnet (FOV 1), the useable homogeneous FOV of the short magnet (FOV 2) is constrained by the shorter magnet design – at least in the longitudinal direction. This has consequences for whole-body MRI. The sketch is not true to scale.

With a length of 125 cm, the magnet lies significantly below the dimensions of the standard systems described above, and the distortion-free useable FOV is also smaller with approx. 30–40 cm (dependent on the application) (Fig. 1.10). The multistation techniques certainly represent an alternative here for the acquisition of larger structures; however, the full potential for exploiting the temporal efficiency of data acquisition tends to lie with the application of the MDS techniques. This much speculation can be made at this juncture: Through the use of MDS techniques, it is potentially possible to further reduce the magnet length and therefore the length of the useable FOV and still carry out whole-body MRI. Taking this thought experiment to its extreme: for axial data acquisition [33, 37, 38] combined with MDS techniques [39], the acquisition of a single homogeneous section should be sufficient to image the entire body as a stack of sections.

1.6   Conclusion

The introduction of whole-body MRI to radiological diagnostics not only has an impact on the hardware and software architecture, data acquisition and image reconstruction, but furthermore on the entire field of image postprocessing, on the presentation of data, and ultimately on the assessment and archiving of greater and ever more comprehensive quantities of images. PACS data archiving systems are becoming increasingly indispensable. The development of algorithms for "Computer-Aided Diagnosis" (CAD) to support radiologists with their examination reporting also contributes to this trend. A paradigm shift has taken place which impacts all the areas described and opens up further indications and attractive applications for MRI.

Bibliography

1. Ho KY, Leiner T, de Haan MW, Kessels AG, Kitslaar PJ, van Engelshoven JM. Peripheral vascular tree stenoses: evaluation with moving-bed infusion-tracking MR angiography. Radiology 1998; 206: 683–92.
2. Wang Y, Lee HM, Khilnani NM, Jagust MB, Winchester PA, Bush HL, Sos TA, Sostman HD. Boluschase MR digital subtraction angiography in the lower extremity. Radiology 1998; 207: 263–9.
3. Meaney JF, Ridgway JP, Chakraverty S, Robertson I, Kessel D, Radjenovic A, Kouwenhoven M, Kassner A, Smith MA. Stepping-table gadolinium-enhanced digital subtraction MR angiography of the aorta and lower extremity arteries: preliminary experience. Radiology 1998; 211: 59–67.
4. Ruehm SG, Hany TF, Pfammatter T, Schneider E, Ladd M, Debatin JF. Pelvic and lower extremity arterial imaging: diagnostic performance of three-dimensional contrast-enhanced MR angiography. AJR Am J Roentgenol 2000; 174(4): 1127–35.
5. Leiner T, Ho KY, Nelemans PJ, de Haan MW, van Engelshoven JM. Three-dimensional contrast-enhanced moving-bed infusion-tracking (MoBI-track) peripheral MR angiography with flexible choice of imaging parameters for each field of view. J Magn Reson Imaging 2000; 11(4): 368–77.
6. Goyen M, Ruehm SG, Barkhausen J, Kroger K, Ladd ME, Truemmler KH, Bosk S, Requardt M, Reykowski A, Debatin JF. Improved multi-station peripheral MR angiography with a dedicated vascular coil. J Magn Reson Imaging 2001; 13(3): 475–80.
7. Ho KY, Leiner T, de Haan MW, van Engelshoven JM. Peripheral MR angiography. Eur Radiol 1999; 9(9): 1765–74.

8. Busch HP, Hoffmann HG, Rock J, Schneider C. MR angiography of pelvic and leg vessels with automatic table movement technique ("MobiTrak"): Clinical experience with 450 studies. RoFo Fortschr Röntgenstr 2001; 173: 405–9.

9. Huber A, Scheidler J, Wintersperger B, Baur A, Schmidt M, Requardt M, Holzknecht N, Helmberger T, Billing A, Reiser M. Moving-table MR angiography of the peripheral runoff vessels: comparison of body coil and dedicated phased array coil systems. AJR Am J Roentgenol 2003; 180(5): 1365–73.

10. Leiner T, Nijenhuis RJ, Maki JH, Lemaire E, Hoogeveen R, van Engelshoven JM. Use of a three-station phased array coil to improve peripheral contrast-enhanced magnetic resonance angiography. J Magn Reson Imaging 2004; 20(3): 417–25.

11. Ruehm SG, Goyen M, Barkhausen J, Kroger K, Bosk S, Ladd ME, Debatin JF. Rapid magnetic resonance angiography for detection of atherosclerosis. Lancet. 2001; 357(9262): 1086–9.

12. Shetty AN, Bis KG, Duerinckx AJ, Narra VR. Lower extremity MR angiography: universal retrofitting of high-field-strength systems with stepping kinematic imaging platforms initial experience. Radiology 2002; 222(1): 284–91.

13. Ruehm SG, Goyen M, Quick HH, Schleputz M, Schleputz H, Bosk S, Barkhausen J, Ladd ME, Debatin JF. [Whole-body MRA on a rolling table platform (AngioSURF)] Rofo Fortschr Röntgenstr 2000; 172(8): 670–4.

14. Goyen M, Quick HH, Debatin JF, Ladd ME, Barkhausen J, Herborn CU, Bosk S, Kuehl H, Schleputz M, Ruehm SG. Whole-body three-dimensional MR angiography with a rolling table platform: initial clinical experience. Radiology 2002; 224(1): 270–7.

15. Winterer JT, Strecker R, Lohrmann C, Schaefer O, Ghanem N, Bley T, Kotter E, Lehnhardt S, Hennig J. Background suppression using magnetization preparation for contrast-enhanced 3D MR angiography of the pelvic and lower leg arteries. Rofo 2003; 175(1): 28–31.

16. Quick HH, Vogt FM, Maderwald S, Herborn CU, Bosk S, Gohde S, Debatin JF, Ladd ME. High spatial resolution whole-body MR angiography featuring parallel imaging: initial experience. RoFo Fortschr Röntgenstr 2004; 176(2): 163–9.

17. Herborn CU, Goyen M, Quick HH, Bosk S, Massing S, Kroeger K, Stoesser D, Ruehm SG, Debatin JF. Whole-body 3D MR angiography of patients with peripheral arterial occlusive disease. AJR Am J Roentgenol 2004; 182(6): 1427–34.

18. Lauenstein TC, Freudenberg LS, Goehde SC, Ruehm SG, Goyen M, Bosk S, Debatin JF, Barkhausen J. Whole-body MRI using a rolling table platform for the detection of bone metastases. Eur Radiol. 2002; 12(8): 2091–9.

19. Lauenstein TC, Goehde SC, Herborn CU, Treder W, Ruehm SG, Debatin JF, Barkhausen J. Threedimensional volumetric interpolated breath-hold MR imaging for whole-body tumor staging in less than 15 minutes: a feasibility study. AJR Am J Roentgenol 2002; 179(2): 445–9.

20. Lauenstein TC, Goehde SC, Herborn CU, Goyen M, Oberhoff C, Debatin JF, Ruehm SG, Barkhausen J. Whole-body MR imaging: evaluation of patients for metastases. Radiology 2004; 233(1): 139–48.

21. Ghanem N, Kelly T, Altehoefer C, Winterer J, Schafer O, Bley TA, Moser E, Langer M. [Wholebody MRI in comparison to skeletal scintigraphy for detection of skeletal metastases in patients with solid tumors][Article in German] Radiologe 2004; 44(9): 864–73.

22. Ruehm SG, Goehde SC, Goyen M. Whole body MR angiography screening. Int J Cardiovasc Imaging 2004; 20(6): 587–91.

23. Goehde SC, Hunold P, Vogt FM, Ajaj W, Goyen M, Herborn CU, Forsting M, Debatin JF, Ruehm SG. Full-body cardiovascular and tumor MRI for early detection of disease: feasibility and initial experience in 298 subjects. AJR Am J Roentgenol 2005; 184(2): 598–611.

24. Johnson KMR, Leavitt GD, Kayser HWM. Total-Body MR imaging in as little as 18 seconds. Radiology 1997; 202: 262–7.].

25. Barkhausen J, Quick HH, Lauenstein T, Goyen M, Ruehm SG, Laub G, Debatin JF, Ladd ME. Whole-body MR imaging in 30 seconds with real-time true FISP and a continuously rolling table platform: feasibility study. Radiology 2001; 220(1): 252–6.

26. Dietrich O, Hajnal JV. Extending the coverage of true volume scans by continuous movement of the subject. ISMRM, 7th Scientific Meeting and Exhibition, Philadelphia, 1999; p. 1653.
27. Kruger DG, Riederer SJ, Grimm RC, Rossman PJ. Continuously moving table data acquisition method for long FOV contrast-enhanced MRA and whole-body MRI. Magn Reson Med 2002; 47(2): 224–31.
28. Zhu Y, Dumoulin CL. Extended field-of-view imaging with table translation and frequency sweeping. Magn Reson Med 2003; 49(6): 1106–12.
29. Fain SB, Browning FJ, Polzin JA, Du J, Zhou Y, Block WF, Grist TM, Mistretta CA. Floating table isotropic projection (FLIPR) acquisition: a time-resolved 3D method for extended field-of-view MRI during continuous table motion. Magn Reson Med 2004; 52(5): 1093–102.
30. Madhuranthakam AJ, Kruger DG, Riederer SJ, Glockner JF, Hu HH. Time-resolved 3D contrastenhanced MRA of an extended FOV using continuous table motion. Magn Reson Med 2004; 51(3): 568–76.
31. Kruger DG, Riederer SJ, Polzin JA, Madhuranthakam AJ, Hu HH, Glockner JF. Dual-velocity continuously moving table acquisition for contrast-enhanced peripheral magnetic resonance angiography. Magn Reson Med 2005; 53(1): 110–7.
32. Polzin JA, Kruger DG, Gurr DH, Brittain JH, Riederer SJ. Correction for gradient nonlinearity in continuously moving table MR imaging. Magn Reson Med 2004; 52(1): 181–7.
33. Zenge MO, Quick HH, Vogt FM, Ladd ME. MR imaging with a continuously rolling table platform and high-precision position feedback. ISMRM, 12th Scientific Meeting and Exhibition, Kyoto, 2004; p. 2381.
34. Zenge MO, Ladd ME, Vogt F, Brauck K, Joekel M, Barkhausen J, Kannengiesser S, Quick HH. High-resolution continuously acquired peripheral MRA featuring self-calibrated parallel imaging. ISMRM, 13th Scientific Meeting and Exhibition, Miami-Beach, 2005; p. 375.
35. Vogt FM, Zenge MO, Ladd ME, Brauck K, Massing S, Barkhausen J, Quick HH. Continuously acquired moving table peripheral MRA compared to conventional multi-station peripheral MRA. ISMRM, 13th Scientific Meeting and Exhibition, Miami-Beach, 2005; p. 455.
36. Keupp J, Aldefeld B, Bornert P. Continuously moving table SENSE imaging. Magn Reson Med 2005; 53(1): 217–20.
37. Shankaranarayanan A, Herfkens R, Hargreaves BM, Polzin JA, Santos JM, Brittain JH. Helical MR: continuously moving table axial imaging with radial acquisitions. Magn Reson Med 2003; 50(5): 1053–60.
38. Scheffler K. Fast volume coverage using sliding, nonuniform angular sampling: the spiral CT approach with projection FLASH and true FISP sequences. In: Proc 9th Scientific Meeting ISMRM, Glasgow, 2001; p. 1774.
39. Fautz HP, Kannengiesser S. Segmented multi-slice (SMS) acquisition for minimum z-FOV axial continuously moving table MRI. In: Proc 13th Scientific Meeting ISMRM, Miami, 2005; p. 2369.

2 Postprocessing and viewing of large MR whole-body data sets

Joachim Graessner

2.1 Data quantities

Besides the challenges in the measurement process, whole-body imaging is also facing considerable demands in postprocessing, evaluation and documentation of very large data sets.

The following overview (Table 2.1) illustrates the enormous growth in data in whole-body imaging compared with conventional single station examinations:

Table 2.1 Average numbers of images in routine MR and whole-body imaging

Examination	Images acquired	Images to be evaluated	Contrasts
Head	~ 120–200	=	T1, T2, Flair, diffusion, post CA T1
Spinal cord	~ 70–90	=	T1, T2, post CA T1
Liver	~ 200–300	=	T1, T2, dyn T1, T1 FS
Pelvis	~ 80–140	=	T1, T2
Knee	~ 100–150	=	T1, PD/T2 FS + (3D)
Peripheral MRA	~ 450	9–30 MIPs + Source	Pre/post CA
Heart	~ 1000	< 1000	Cine, perfusion, late enhancement
Whole-body	> 2000	~ 2000	div. + partial-body (liver, heart) scans

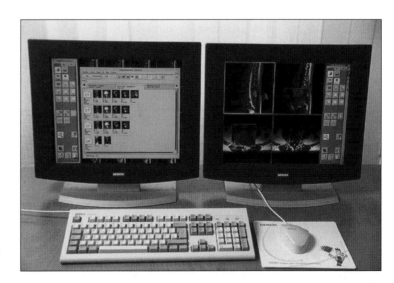

Figure 2.1 Dual-monitor workstation.

Table 2.2 Protocol structure for a 6-station metastasis search and a 5-station MR angio

Table movement 205 ipat	Size 205-5 steps
I_scout	Scout-head-neck-0mm
I_t2_tse_tra_head	Vessel-Head
I_t1_fl2d_op_ph_sag_c-sp	Scout-thorax-380mm
I_t2_tirm_cor_mbh	Scout-Abdomen-760mm
II_scout_280_F	Vessel-Abdomen-760mm
II_t1_fl2d_op_ph_sag_t-sp	Scout-upper-leg-1140mm
II_t2_tirm_cor_mbh	Vessel-upperleg-1140mm
III_scout_560_F	Scout-lower-leg-1520mm
III_t1_fl2d_op_ph_sag_l-sp	TFL-cor-CareBolus
III_t2_tirm_cor_mbh	FI3d_cor_Head-0mm
IV_scout_840_F	FI3d_cor_Thorax-380mm
V_t2_tirm_cor	FI3d_cor_Abdomen-760mm
VI_scout_1120_F	FI3d_cor_upper-leg-1140mm
VI_t2_tirm_cor	FI3d_cor_lower-leg-1520mm
VI_scout_1400_F	Injection+rerun_Carebolus
VI_t2_tirm_cor	

The increase in the number of relevant images for a report by a factor of 10–20 compared with conventional MR examinations requires a specific viewing and postprocessing strategy dependent on the particular investigation.

For evaluation during ongoing examinations, scrolling within the measured series is generally the only feasible option. The number of series can easily exceed 40 depending on the examination.

Comparison with any potential pre-examinations that may have been performed is straightforward with the parallel screen layout of one or more monitors. Length, area and volume changes of lesions can be determined effectively with this method.

Series evaluation will remain the standard even for whole-body examinations, with added partial-body detail scans for brain, heart, liver and joints.

Table 2.2 shows measurement programs for a whole-body MR metastasis screening examination that are still relatively short (coronal orientation incl. sagittal T1 spine and transverse T2 head as well as a whole-body angiography):

Aside from the main measurements, both program examples include 5 and 9 auxiliary measurements, respectively, for the basic localizer (scout) for each table position. The simple metastasis search itself generates 10 series; a whole-body MR angiography on 5 stations produces 10 series, as well as the automatically generated MIP series on the subtracted series at each station. A combination of both programs, or supplementary T1 measurements before and after contrast agent (CA) administration, reduces the number of auxiliary measurements required, but leads to a further increase in the quantity of series to be evaluated [7].

A more complex procedure for screening in Table 2.3 shows the integration of additional organ-specific measurements also for transverse slices:

The program in Table 2.3 alone produces 22 main series plus 7 auxiliary series. Integration of additional measurements for the heart and vascular system, the colon, and the large joints is currently undergoing evaluation in extensive clinical studies [1]. Although the measurement time for the comprehensive whole-body studies is about 1 hour or more, times of less than 15 minutes are attainable for specific investigations such as metastasis

Table 2.3 Protocol structure for an example of a 5-station screening program (T1, T2, and STIR)

high_res_ipat2	III_haste_cor_448_p2
I_scout_head-neck	III_t1_tse_cor_384_p2
I_t2_tirm_cor_384_pat2	__Pelvis__
I_t2_haste_cor_448_p2	III_t2_tse_tra_384_pelvis
I_t1_tse_cor_384_pat2	IV_scout_1060 feet
I_t2_tirm_tra_da-flu_head	IV_t2_tirm_cor_384_p2
II_scout_280_feet_tho-abd	IV_haste_cor_448_p2
II_t2_tirm_cor_384_pat2	IV_t1_tse_cor_384_p2
II_t2_haste_cor_mbh_448_p2	V_scout_1400 feet
II_t1_tse_cor_384_pat2	V_t2_tirm_cor_384_pat2
__Lung metastasis__	V_haste_cor_448_p2
II_t2_tirm_tra_mbh_320_p2	V_t1_tse_cor_384_pat2
__Abdomen__	_Cervical and thoracic spine_
II_t1_fl2d_fs_tra_mbh_p2	localizer_80_F
II_t2_tse_fs_tra_ga_320_p2	t2_tirm_sag_pat2
III_scout_680 feet_pelvis	_thoracic and lumbar spine_
III_t2_tirm_cor_384_p2	localizer_390_F
	t2_tirm_sag_pat2

search [2]; pure whole-body MR angiography programs may be realized in less than 5 min. [3].

The consequent use of parallel imaging techniques reduces measurement times further to much less than one hour, even for comprehensive whole-body programs [5, 6, 8].

2.2 Data reduction and workflow

MR angiography of peripheral vessels with a 2- to 4-station technique has shown that the large number of images and series remains manageable due to the reduction of information in maximum intensity projections (MIP) and subtraction series of pre and post CA measurements. Station by station viewing of the source images in the regions of suspicion is still essential [4].

In examinations including the heart, a virtual reduction of data is possible through the cine view of the functional series by viewing the images with fast scrolling, which gives rise to a correspondingly reduced evaluation time.

The quantity of data in certain MR measurement techniques can always be cut down through integrated (Inline®) or through manual processing. The processing of images integrated into measurement protocols frequently relieves the user of time-consuming postprocessing, consequently improving the entire workflow, with measurement and reporting taking center stage.

As with the angiography data sets described above, the reduction of data helps in the initial viewing of the image material or to document quantitative results. Nevertheless, the individual images usually have to be inspected.

Of the techniques listed in Table 2.4, subtraction, MIP, ADC image, and, above all, composing are of major significance.

Composing offers the option of linking morphological measurements of the same contrast at different overlapping table positions to form a single image. The program automatically performs the necessary distortion correction over large measurement fields and

Table 2.4 Processing and postprocessing to reduce the quantity of data (selection)

	Technique	Measurement method/ input data	Result	Reduction	Inline[1]
1	Subtraction	Pre/post CA T1 series Pre/post CA MR angio	Enrichment image Vessel data set	2:1	X X
2	Standard deviation N images	Phase contrast MRA Dynamic MRA Pulsatile flow	Emphasis of dynamic changes	N:1	X X X
3	MIP	Angio data	Vessel image	> 80–100:1	X
3	t-test	BOLD measurements	Activation map	> 60:1	X
5	ADC	Diffusion weighting	ADC map	3:1	X
6	Time-to-peak	Brain perfusion	Perfusion map	~ 50:1	X
7	Wash in/out	Mamma perfusion	Emphasis on fast CA uptake and washout	6–10:1	X
8	Composing	Morphological and angio data sets for different table positions	Overall image with interpolation in the overlapping regions	2–8:1	X
9	Dyn. signal analysis	Heart perfusion	Standardized curves	~40:1	
10	Volume determination	Heart function	Tables	~ 250:1	

1. i.e. processing is already defined and performed in the measurement protocol

offers a suggestion for the combination of the respective stations. Manual shifting of the overlap zone is possible. Synchronous scrolling of 2 series with different contrasts is also achievable, either in the overview mode or in a detail zoom with movable magnifying glass function (Fig. 2.2–2.4).

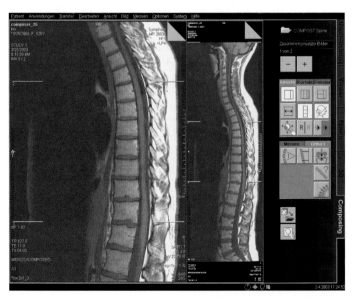

Figure 2.2 Composing a 3-station spinal column T1 scan; detail and overall view.

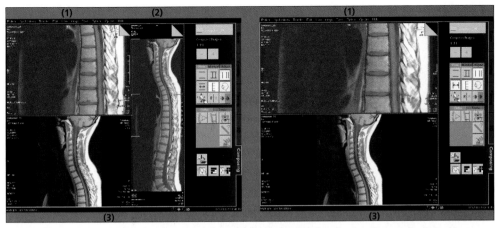

Figure 2.3 Composing with the example of a spinal column for detail, overview and original images: (1) detail image, (2) overview image, (3) original image.

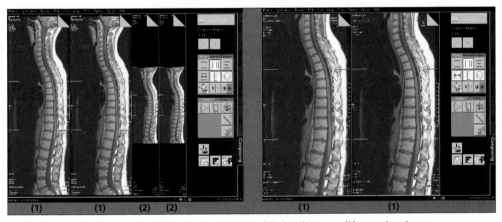

Figure 2.4 Composing with 2 comparison segments: (1) detail image, (2) overview image.

Syngo Composing task card: The sagittal image was compiled from 3 individual images at different table positions. The overlap zones were calculated with smoothing interpolation (at the level of the horizontal marking lines). The user navigates through the entire image stack of a composite series and can zoom into target regions. It is possible to measure distances, kyphosis and scoliosis angles as well as height differences. Storage of the composed images in DICOM format reduces the number of series to be shown for a subsequent demonstration of the images.

Figure 2.3 shows a layout which, besides the total overview, also shows the original data and enlarged detail images in a working map. Marking and labeling of pathological findings with subsequent storage of these extracted images serves to accelerate the final report.

A comparative depiction of previous and new examinations or of different contrasts and orientations may be seen in Figures 2.4 and 2.5. Synchronous scrolling or zooming makes comparison of the images easier.

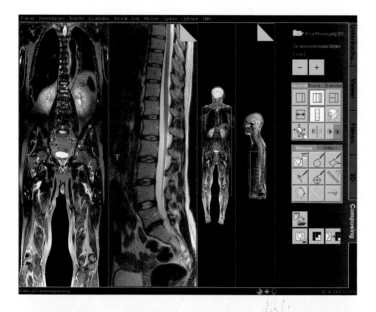

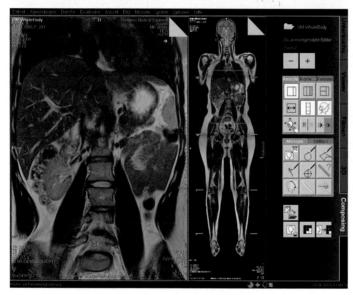

Figure 2.5a, b 2 orientations in parallel configuration; whole-body image with liver zoom.

2.3   Outlook

Composing can be helpful for the demonstration of data and also for a comprehensive overview. Nevertheless, process-controlled diagnostic procedures will be required in the future, which, similar to the CT software shown in Figure 2.6 for coin lesion marking in the lung, provide the radiologist with tools for marking and extracting results in order to add the essential image segments taken from the wealth of image data to the final report or a structured report in accordance with the DICOM standard.

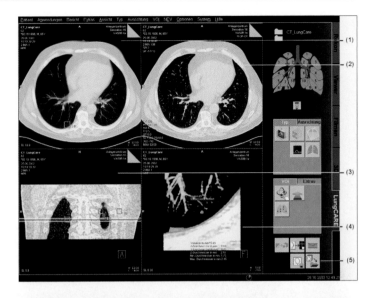

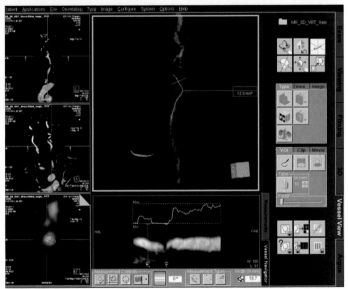

Figure 2.6 CT of the lung, CARE software for determining coin lesions; vessel-view map for mapping the midline of vessel sections and determining the degree of stenosis.

Segmental viewing of the data is still necessary. Cross-referencing with correlated mouse pointers simplifies orientation on series with different section orientation; the prerequisite is that the data sets have a common coordinate system. This means that the data from a session are acquired with automatic table movement and without patient repositioning.

New programs, such as COLON processing, which can use both CT and MR images as input data, today offer the possibility of marking results in the software interface to generate structured reports. This approach to viewing image data and the extraction of the relevant images and data will be further expanded to cope with large data sets.

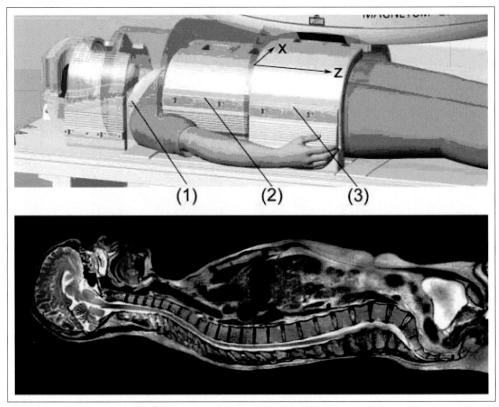

Figure 2.7 Patient set-up with a vertical field of 0.35 T with local coils: (1) CP Head/Neck Array Coil with Neck Coil, medium, (2) Body/Spine Array Coil, medium, (3) Body/Spine Array Coil, large.

Other software modules, such as the „vesselview" program shown in Figure 2.6, allow processing the midline of suspicious sections of tortuous vessels, allowing a non-overlapping rotation around the mid-axis and determination of degree of stenosis. In this way, 80–128 sections and more of a contrast-enhanced MR angiography series can be evaluated compressed in one view port.

In contrast to computed tomography (CT) with its water-referenced Houndfield units, the intensity images generated in MRI are less well discriminating for different tissue types and are therefore less well suited for computer-assisted algorithms (CAD). Systems based on suggestions for the user, e.g. for STIR sequences, are conceivable.

Figure 2.7 shows that at low field strengths (0.35 T) there are also at least partial-body multistation applications with dedicated array coils.

In conclusion, it can be said that whole-body MRI, similar to multi-slice CT, generates a large volume of work for the radiologist, although the morphological series (STIR, T1, T2) can be evaluated even during the patient examination as a result of the sequential nature of the measurements. A preliminary or conclusive result can therefore be presented very soon after the end of the completed examination.

Bibliography

1. Goehde SC, Hunold P, Vogt FM, Ajaj W, Goyen M, Herborn CU, Forsting M, Debatin JF, Ruehm SG. Full-body cardiovascular and tumor MRI for early detection of disease: feasibility and initial experience in 298 subjects; AJR Am J Roentgenol 2005 Feb; 184(2): 598–611.
2. Lauenstein TC, Goehde SC, Herborn CU, Goyen M, Oberhoff C, Debatin JF, Ruehm SG, Barkhausen J. Whole-body MR imaging: evaluation of patients for metastases. Radiology 2004 Oct; 233(1): 139–48
3. Herborn CU, Goyen M, Quick HH, Bosk S, Massing S, Kroeger K, Stoesser D, Ruehm SG, Debatin JF. Whole-body 3D MR angiography of patients with peripheral arterial occlusive disease. AJR Am J Roentgenol 2004 Jun; 182(6): 1427–34.
4. Fenchel M, Requardt M, Tomaschko K, Kramer U, Stauder NI, Naegele T, Schlemmer HP, Claussen CD, Miller S. Whole-body MR angiography using a novel 32-receiving-channel MR system with surface coil technology: first clinical experience; J Magn Reson Imaging 2005 May; 21(5): 596–603.
5. Schlemmer HP, Schafer J, Pfannenberg C, Radny P, Korchidi S, Muller-Horvat C, Nagele T, Tomaschko K, Fenchel M, Claussen CD. Fast whole-body assessment of metastatic disease using a novel magnetic resonance imaging system: initial experiences. Invest Radiol 2005 Feb; 40(2): 64–71.
6. Kramer H, Schoenberg SO, Nikolaou K, Huber A, Struwe A, Winnik E, Wintersperger B, Dietrich O, Kiefer B, Reiser MF. Cardiovascular whole body MRI with parallel imaging. Radiologe 2004 Sep; 44(9): 835–43.
7. Lenk S, Fischer S, Kotter I, Claussen CD, Schlemmer HP. Possibilities of whole-body MRI for investigating musculoskeletal diseases. Radiologe 2004 Sep; 44(9): 844–53.
8. Schafer JF, Fischmann A, Lichy M, Vollmar J, Fenchel M, Claussen CD, Schlemmer HP. Oncologic screening with whole-body MRI: possibilities and limitations. Radiologe 2004 Sep; 44(9): 854–63.

Clinical Applications

Christoph U. Herborn

Atherosclerosis is a complex systematic disease affecting the arterial bed of the human body, and even at a young age it leads to verifiable changes in the vessel wall. These typically include thickening of the vessel wall, as well as the formation of circumscribed plaque in flow regions which are subject to special hemodynamic stress. These are in particular branching structures or long straight sections of arteries, such as the bifurcation of the carotid arteries, the origin of the renal arteries, the aortic bifurcation, and the passage of the femoral artery in the adductor canal in the thigh. Atherosclerotic changes in the coronary arteries are of particular relevance, as these arteries, being end arteries, show insufficient collaterals in their supply region.

For patients with relevant atherosclerotic vascular changes in the lower extremities, additional wall changes are often verifiable in other vessels [1], which are clinically proven to increase the likelihood of other complaints. However, these complaints are often concealed through the dominance of the primary symptoms (e.g. severe chest pain with coronary heart disease or transitory ischemic attacks with symptomatic stenosis of the internal carotid artery, each with accompanying, but as yet undiscovered, peripheral arterial occlusive disease) due to limited physical stamina and are only discovered through dedicated investigation and examinations.

Extensive imaging techniques to examine the entire arterial vascular system are therefore indicated to systematically detect and hence quantify the manifestation of atherosclerosis. Digital subtraction angiography (DSA) permits selective and superposition-free depiction of nearly all vascular territories of the human body. Besides determining the nature, distribution and relevance of atherosclerotic vascular changes, the technique offers the advantage, using a vascular introducer sheath into the arterial vessel system and the insertion of special catheters, of combining diagnosis and therapy in a single examination and of treating the relevant region of disease with circumscribed dilation or the targeted insertion of stents. Despite these options, because of the overall X-ray dosage and the limited quantity of iodine-based X-ray contrast agent that can be used due to its renal toxicology, the use of DSA is not practicable for routine whole-body angiography. Due to its invasiveness and the associated risks, it is also excluded from the outset as a method for screening purposes or for screening examinations.

The latest advancement in computed tomography (CT) to multislice devices with up to 64 detector lines allows selective and precise imaging of the arterial vessels from head to foot within a few seconds thanks to the temporal coordination of contrast agent administration with data acquisition. Despite its high spatial and temporal resolution, image analysis of CT angiography is limited by laborious postprocessing. Calcified vessel regions particularly present problems here, because precise quantification of the constriction of the vessel lumen is only possible to a limited extent as a result of the hardening artifacts in X-ray radiation. In addition, for both CT and DSA, not only does the total X-ray dosage play a role for the patient, but the potential renal damage from the contrast agent used must also be taken into consideration. It is therefore understandable that DSA and CT are mainly used today to depict selected vascular territories, and both techniques are limited in achieving a comprehensive vascular clinical picture by their segmental applicability.

The introduction of magnetic resonance angiography (MRA) using paramagnetic contrast agents in radiological diagnostics at the beginning of the 1990s laid the foundations of non-invasive, fast, and safe examination methods with which we can today depict large vascular territories in a few moments with high temporal and spatial resolution [2–6]. Initially, the early enhancement of the surrounding soft tissue and the maximum permissible amount of contrast agent stood in the way of using MRI for vascular imaging; also, a length of only up to just under 50 cm in the field of examination could be covered. The recent introduction of new and above all ultra-fast gradient systems, combined with bolus tracking techniques with fast table movement after injection of a single contrast agent bolus, allows imaging of several vascular territories in rapid succession. Whereas at first the depiction of the abdominal aorta through to the lower legs was possible during a single examination, gadolinium contrast-enhanced MR angiography of the blood vessels from head to foot is now possible in less than a minute with the latest generation of MR scanners [7–10]. The correlation of this image material with DSA examinations has produced very good agreement between the methods, so that the expansion of the examination region from circumscribed vessel regions to the entire vascular system has opened up the way for a paradigm shift in imaging: the all-encompassing evaluation of a complex clinical picture with a single, non-invasive examination (Fig. 3.1). On the basis of whole-body MRA, therapeutic options for symptomatic patients can be discussed and optimally planned, while the methods can also be applied in the healthy population as part of a health screening program to detect clinically inert early stages of atherosclerosis and thereby support preventive measures (see Chap. 12).

The whole-body MR angiography concept is today based on two methods: Firstly, the acquisition of five slightly overlapping 3D data sets in immediate succession using a manually positionable moving table technique [10–15]. The first data set covers the aortic arch, as well as the supraaortal vessels including the carotid arteries; the second data set images the abdominal aorta with its visceral branches, as well as the renal arteries. The pelvic arteries are acquired in the third data set, and the last two data sets present the arteries in the upper and lower legs. The acquisition time for each individual 3D data set is 12 seconds; the examination table is moved manually between the respective stations during each of the 3-second-long pauses. For 5 stations, a total acquisition time of 72 seconds results for the head to foot examination.

For the examination, the patient is placed on a rolling table platform (Angiography System for Unlimited Rolling Field of Views, Angio*SURF*, MR-Innovation GmbH, Essen, Germany, see Chap. 1), which is mounted on a roller system on the original patient table and allows examination with a surface coil system (phased array coils). The surface coil increases the signal-to-noise ratio (SNR) compared with the body coil and improves spatial resolution, which for the described protocol is defined with an effective interpolated voxel size of 0.8×0.8×2 mm. This leads to improved discrimination, especially of the smaller vessels of the lower legs.

For planning the examination itself, overview images are firstly taken of the five regions (moving vessel scout protocol: 6 slices per station, TR: 539 ms, TE: 10 ms, TI: 300 ms, flip

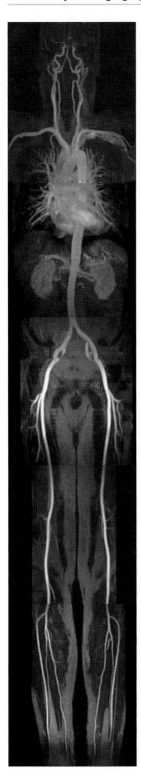

angle: 50°, slice thickness: 8 mm, matrix: 114×256, field of view: 400 mm, acquisition time: 20 seconds). The time of passage of the contrast agent from the lower arm to the descending aorta to the level of the base of the heart is then determined. For this purpose, a test bolus of 2 ml gadolinium is injected at a speed of 1.3 ml/s into the cubital vein and flushed with a physiological saline solution at the same injection speed. An axial, multiphase turboFlash sequence is used for this purpose. It allows a temporal resolution of 1 image/s.

The acquisition of 3D data sets to depict the arterial vascular system is performed with a fast gradient-echo sequence. A total of five data sets with an overlap of 3 cm are acquired, so that a total length of 176 cm can be covered using Angio*SURF*. If required, the examination area can be extended to six stations to enlarge the field of examination. In contrast to the examination of patients with peripheral arterial occlusive disease, screening examinations do not require the acquisition of native (non-contrast-enhanced) data sets to produce subtractions on account of the very short repetition times with good background signal suppression.

A second method does not use a single surface coil under which the patient is moved, but rather covers the body from head to foot with several surface coils, each optimized for the respective region of examination [16]. During the examination, the patient is automatically moved between a total of four stations to complete image acquisition at the isocenter of the magnet at each station. An area can be covered over a length of 205 cm. The latest MR systems allow the combination of up to 76 different coil elements (matrix coils) and data acquisition with up to 32 receiver channels operating simultaneously (see Chap. 1). As a result, an optimal spatial resolution in the submillimeter range is achieved for each station, and a maximum signal strength from the tissue examined is measured.

Both techniques can be optimized by using parallel imaging; this allows a significant reduction in the acquisition time with unchanged spatial resolution. On the other hand, the spatial resolution of the examination can be considerably improved with parallel imaging without longer acquisition times. In parallel imaging, the spatially distributed MR signal is picked up

Figure 3.1 Whole-body MRA is suitable not only for the evaluation of the vessel status of the patient with clinical symptoms of PAOD, but it can also be applied as part of a screening examination for patients with an elevated risk of arterial vascular bed diseases. The absence of risks, good tolerance of the contrast agents used, short examination times, and both high temporal and spatial resolution depiction of vessels makes whole-body MRA an ideal technical tool for the comprehensive cardiovascular check-up.

from various receiver coils. All coil elements used for MRA can be exploited for performing parallel imaging in all three spatial planes. Varying MR spatial signal intensities are received simultaneously from these receiver coils with different spatial intensity profiles. The number of phase-encoding steps can therefore be reduced, without the spatial resolution or the matrix size of the image having to be restricted. The wrap-around artifacts that possibly arise in conventional image reconstruction are corrected with the parallely-acquired data and the individually adapted coil profiles of the receiver elements. Data reconstruction can be performed both in the computed image (sensitivity encoding, SENSE) [17], as well as in k-space (SMASH) [18, 19]. While the technique was initially not possible for whole-body applications, the latest algorithms, with an autocalibration measurement in each sequence for the respective coil configuration, permit an arbitrary number of coil elements and therefore also table movement between the respective stations with optimal signal processing (Tim: total imaging matrix, Siemens Medical Solutions, Erlangen, Germany), making them especially suitable for MR angiography of larger or composite vessel territories. Parallel imaging can also be applied using a single receiver coil (with several elements) and the table movement technique [20]. The reduced signal, which can lead to a compromise in image quality compared with conventional acquisition techniques, represents a limitation for parallel imaging techniques.

A technique to improve image quality, which was evaluated at the beginning of clinical MRA, has recently been rediscovered and is of special interest for users of systems that cannot be equipped with parallel imaging: subsystolic venous compression for improved arterial vessel presentation. Whereas the initial investigations were still aimed at improving the examination quality of individual vessel stations in the lower leg [21], the successful use of transient venous compression (VENCO) has also proved convincing for MRA of the extremities and whole-body MRA [22, 23]. Before the contrast agent is injected, blood pressure cuffs are applied on both thighs and are inflated to a constant pressure of approx. 40–60 mm Hg. This pressure is maintained throughout the entire examination. The venous stasis thus produced slows down the flow of contrast agent from the arterial vessel bed and thereby allows a longer imaging window with improved spatial resolution and consequently better image quality and diagnostic validity.

For all of the examination techniques described, the contrast agent is applied biphasically with an automatic injector (e.g. MR Spectris, Medrad, Pittsburgh/USA; Ulrich Medizintechnik, Ulm, Germany). The total dose used is 0.2 mmol/kg body weight. The first half of the dose is injected with a flow rate of 1.3 ml/s, the second half with a flow rate of 0.7 ml/s, followed by 30 ml saline solution with a flow rate of 1.3 ml/s. By reducing the flow rate to 0.7 ml/s for the second half of the contrast agent injection, possible venous superposition of the lower extremity arterial vessels is avoided. The examination time for whole-body MRA using Angio*SURF* is approx. 10 min including repositioning the patient and breathing instructions – roughly the same as whole-body MRA with several coils, which have to be precisely located during preparation. The evaluation of the image data takes place in both cases at a digital station.

The biphasic injection allows data acquisition of the first two stations (skull and thorax/upper abdomen) during an initial high flow rate (1.3 ml/s), whereas a slower flow rate (0.7 ml/s) is used for the remaining stations to achieve depiction of the vessels without superposition. Marginal portal venous or peripheral venous contamination hinders image analysis only in maximum intensity projections, whereas appropriate postprocessing can almost completely cancel it out in multi-planar reconstructions.

Whole-body MRA of patients with clinical suspicion of peripheral arterial occlusive disease (PAOD) not only succeeded in detecting or excluding the presence of relevant vascular disease in the suspected peripheral vascular territory, but by capturing additional vessel territories detected in a third of the patients additional relevant vascular changes, which prior to the examination had not been suspected or had only caused intermittent symptoms (Fig. 3.2) [10, 12–14, 24, 25]. Most studies succeeded in comparing and confirming the MR results with those of invasive DSA of the lower extremities; the other vessel territories were verified with supplementary examinations, such as selective MRA or color-encoded duplex sonography. The excellent correlation of whole-body MRA with these methods to detect or exclude atherosclerotic vessel changes in the entire arterial vascular system, combined with relatively short examination times, indicates the potential of this imaging technique for patients with PAOD. The high prevalence of concomitant arterial lesions in patients with peripheral arterial occlusive disease underlines the systemic pattern of atherosclerosis and the resulting arterial occlusive disease. Accordingly, in up to a third of cases, patients with clinically manifest peripheral arterial occlusive disease also

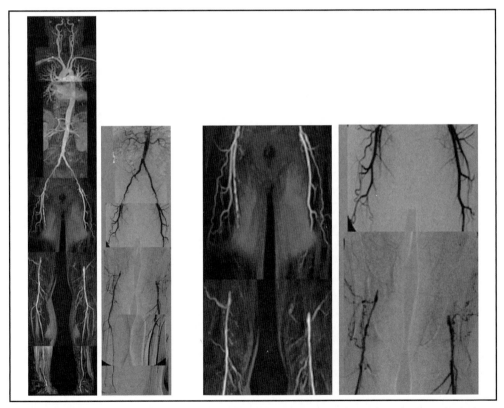

Figure 3.2 The figure shows the excellent correlation between the catheter-based DSA and whole-body MR angiography of a 68-year-old man with peripheral occlusive disease in Fontaine stage IIb and bilateral occlusions of the superficial femoral artery. Whereas DSA is restricted to the lower extremities, the AngioSURF examination also succeeds in imaging the complete arterial vascular system in a true 3D data set without overlay. Here the pathology (enlargement) is precisely captured, which facilitates the subsequent therapy planning (in this case the installation of a bilateral vessel bypass).

have renal artery stenosis [26], and symptomatic changes in the vessels supplying the brain occur in approx. 26 to 50% of cases [27, 28].

Developments towards using single or multiple surface coils combined with fast table movement techniques have overcome the limitations of initial whole-body examinations (weak signal, poor spatial resolution) [7, 8] and today can even image the fine vessels of the lower leg at the level of the ankle mortise with high resolution in routine applications. Besides the improvements in image quality, this development is also reflected in an improvement in diagnostic precision [9, 15, 25]. In selected works, the use of this new technique has led to reports on the sensitivity and specificity in detecting stenotic regions of the arteries of the lower leg of up to 98% [9, 29].

The prevalence of thoracic and abdominal aortic aneurysms in patients with arterial occlusive disease is also known to be elevated [30]. Whereas the use of screening for aortic aneurysms among asymptomatic patients is controversial and there exist a number of varying recommendations in this respect [24–31], there is widespread agreement that targeted examination of the thoracic-abdominal aorta in the patient group with peripheral arterial occlusive disease is justified [35, 36], which further underlines the potential for whole-body MRA with the depiction of the entire course of the aorta and its branches.

Against this background, MRI is also suitable as the imaging screening technique of choice in the detection of cardiovascular diseases in a putatively healthy population (see Chap. 12). The absence of side effects (especially no ionizing radiation), combined with high soft tissue contrast, as well as high spatial and temporal resolution, are ideal prerequisites for use as an imaging technique for screening (Fig. 3.3).

The results presented in the literature to date document the performance of MR angiography in this context [16, 37]. The conditions for performing an examination of this type include optimized technical equipment with high performance hardware, a moving table platform, and an experienced examination team. This also applies for evaluating the data acquired.

The use of various gadolinium-based contrast agents for MR angiography has been described in the literature. Although most MR examinations worldwide are performed with gadopentetate dimeglumine (Gd-DTPA, Magnevist®, Schering, Berlin, Germany), additional compounds have been licensed in recent times, whose use in whole-body MRA appears to be promising [38–41]. Certain preparations remain in the blood pool for a longer period due to transitory bonding of individual molecules to serum albumin and thereby give rise to an enhanced signal (gadobenate dimeglumine, Gd-BOPTA, MultiHance®, Altana Pharma, Konstanz, Germany) [42–45]. A further neutral gadolinium chelate is Gadobutrol (Gadovist®, Schering, Berlin, Germany), which, due to its higher molarity, produces higher relaxivity in the blood and can generate a higher intravascular signal than Gd-DTPA [12, 38, 41]. Further contrast agents will be licensed in the near future, from which an improvement in image quality is to be expected: in addition to other preparations currently under investigation in clinical multi-center studies, Vasovist® (Gadofosveset, MS-325, Schering, Berlin, Germany) is the first intravascular contrast agent approved for use with magnetic resonance angiography in the European Union (Chap. 4). Vasovist® reversibly binds to albumin providing extended intravascular enhancement compared to existing extracellular magnetic resonance contrast agents. The relaxivity of Vasovist® compared with conventional gadolinium compounds is considerably higher [46, 47]. It remains to be seen how the quality of whole-body MRA can be improved with new contrast agents of this type, and whether new vessel territories can be opened up through the use of these preparations; a possible indication exists, for instance, in the imaging of the coronary arteries with MRA after injection of Vasovist®.

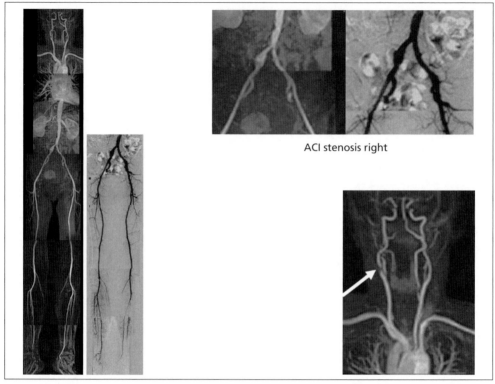

ACI stenosis right

Figure 3.3 Whole-body MRA with Angio*SURF* technology shows the aneurysm of the right common iliac artery with the same diagnostic quality as the invasive DSA examination of this 64-year-old woman with symptoms of PAOD in Fontaine stage IIa. The holistic depiction of the arterial vascular system also revealed a severe stenosis of the right internal carotid artery (arrow), which was confirmed with duplex sonography.

Despite the promising initial results, the technique described in this article is known to have its limitations. In the case of suspected stenosis, the limited spatial resolution of whole-body MRA requires a subsequent dedicated examination to exactly quantify the affected vascular regions, either using color-encoded duplex sonography or DSA, which is still regarded as the standard of reference for vascular assessment. A shift in favor of MR angiography here has become recently apparent, which could ultimately render invasive diagnostic examination superfluous.

Finally, neither the small intracranial vessels nor the coronary arteries are captured in whole-body MRA. Although intracranial blood vessels are rarely affected by atherosclerotic changes in the western world, the supplementation of the examination protocol with time-of-flight MRA without the additional administration of contrast agent and with relatively short acquisition times of just a few minutes could round off the examination in this area. The absence of the adequate depiction of the coronary arteries is far more problematic. These vessels are more frequently and far more relevantly the site of atherosclerosis manifestation, with potentially catastrophic consequences. The evaluation of the coronary arteries is also important because atherosclerotic changes can be effectively treated with minimally-invasive or established operational techniques. The imaging of coronary arteries with MRA techniques, both with and without the use of contrast agents, places enormous demands on the operator and scanner and often still only delivers results of limited conclusiveness and practical value [48, 49]. Therefore, the clinical use of MRA of the coronary vessels for screening to exclude coronary disease is still to be considered a subject of research far remote from clinical routine work.

Summarizing, the three-dimensional contrast-enhanced MR angiography technique presented in this article shows itself to be a reliable technique to image vascular changes in patients with peripheral arterial occlusive disease. Moreover, whole-body imaging of arterial vessels opens up reliable detection of additional and also relevant atherosclerotic vascular regions above the lower extremities of these patients. For this reason, whole-body MRA, which can be performed within an examination time of less than 10 minutes including preparation and positioning of the patient, appears to be suitable as a diagnostic reference technique for the clinical suspicion of hemodynamically-relevant stenoses in the arterial vascular system, as well as an imaging method of choice for the health maintenance of a supposedly vascular-healthy population.

Bibliography

1. American Heart Association. 2004 Heart and stroke statistical update. In: Dallas, Texas: American Heart Association, 2003; 2003.
2. Meaney JF, Weg JG, Chenevert TL, Stafford-Johnson D, Hamilton BH, Prince MR. Diagnosis of pulmonary embolism with magnetic resonance angiography. N Engl J Med 1997; 336: 1422–7.
3. Prince MR. Gadolinium-enhanced MR aortography. Radiology 1994; 191: 155–64.
4. Shellock FG, Kanal E. Safety of magnetic resonance imaging contrast agents. J Magn Reson Imaging 1999; 10: 477–84.
5. Prince MR, Narasimham DL, Stanley JC, Chenevert TL, Williams DM, Marx MV, Cho KJ. Breathhold gadolinium-enhanced MR angiography of the abdominal aorta and its major branches. Radiology 1995; 197: 785–92.
6. Goyen M, Debatin JF, Ruehm SG. Peripheral magnetic resonance angiography. Top Magn Reson Imaging 2001; 12: 327–35.
7. Ho KY, Leiner T, de Haan MW, Kessels AG, Kitslaar PJ, van Engelshoven JM. Peripheral vascular tree stenoses: evaluation with moving-bed infusion-tracking MR angiography. Radiology 1998; 206: 683–92.
8. Meaney JF, Ridgway JP, Chakraverty S, Robertson I, Kessel D, Radjenovic A, Kouwenhoven M, Kassner A, Smith MA. Stepping-table gadolinium-enhanced digital subtraction MR angiography of the aorta and lower extremity arteries: preliminary experience. Radiology 1999; 211: 59–67.
9. Ruehm SG, Hany TF, Pfammatter T, Schneider E, Ladd M, Debatin JF. Pelvic and lower extremity arterial imaging: diagnostic performance of three-dimensional contrast-enhanced MR angiography. AJR Am J Roentgenol 2000; 174: 1127–35.
10. Ruehm SG, Goyen M, Barkhausen J, Kroger K, Bosk S, Ladd ME, Debatin JF. Rapid magnetic resonance angiography for detection of atherosclerosis. Lancet 2001; 357: 1086–91.
11. Ruehm SG, Goyen M, Quick HH, Schleputz M, Schleputz H, Bosk S, Barkhausen J, Ladd ME, Debatin JF. [Whole-body MRA on a rolling table platform (AngioSURF)]. Rofo 2000; 172: 670–4.
12. Herborn CU, Goyen M, Quick HH, Bosk S, Massing S, Kroeger K, Stoesser D, Ruehm SG, Debatin JF. Whole-body 3D MR angiography of patients with peripheral arterial occlusive disease. AJR Am J Roentgenol 2004; 182: 1427–34.
13. Goyen M, Quick HH, Debatin JF, Ladd ME, Barkhausen J, Herborn CU, Bosk S, Kuehl H, Schleputz M, Ruehm SG. Whole-body three-dimensional MR angiography with a rolling table platform: initial clinical experience. Radiology 2002; 224: 270–7.

14. Goyen M, Ruehm SG, Debatin JF. [Arterial vascular screening with whole body MR angiography]. Med Klin 2002; 97: 285–9.

15. Goyen M, Herborn CU, Kroger K, Lauenstein TC, Debatin JF, Ruehm SG. Detection of Atherosclerosis: Systemic Imaging for Systemic Disease with Whole-Body Three-dimensional MR Angiography – Initial Experience. Radiology 2003.

16. Kramer H, Schoenberg SO, Nikolaou K, Huber A, Struwe A, Winnik E, Wintersperger B, Dietrich O, Kiefer B, Reiser MF. [Cardiovascular whole body MRI with parallel imaging]. Radiologe 2004; 44: 835–43.

17. Pruessmann KP, Weiger M, Scheidegger MB, Boesiger P. SENSE: sensitivity encoding for fast MRI. Magn Reson Med 1999; 42: 952–62.

18. Sodickson DK, McKenzie CA, Li W, Wolff S, Manning WJ, Edelman RR. Contrast-enhanced 3D MR angiography with simultaneous acquisition of spatial harmonics: A pilot study. Radiology 2000; 217: 284–9.

19. Goldfarb JW, Holland AE. Parallel magnetic resonance imaging using coils with localized sensitivities. Magn Reson Imaging 2004; 22: 1025–9.

20. Quick HH, Vogt FM, Maderwald S, Herborn CU, Bosk S, Gohde S, Debatin JF, Ladd ME. High spatial resolution whole-body MR angiography featuring parallel imaging: initial experience. Rofo 2004; 176: 163–9.

21. Bilecen D, Schulte AC, Bongartz G, Heidecker HG, Aschwanden M, Jager KA. Infragenual cuffcompression reduces venous contamination in contrast-enhanced MR angiography of the calf. J Magn Reson Imaging 2004; 20: 347–51.

22. Bilecen D, Jager KA, Aschwanden M, Heidecker HG, Schulte AC, Bongartz G. Cuff-compression of the proximal calf to reduce venous contamination in contrast-enhanced stepping-table magnetic Resonance angiography. Acta Radiol 2004; 45: 510–5.

23. Herborn CU, Ajaj W, Goyen M, Massing S, Ruehm SG, Debatin JF. Peripheral vasculature: wholebody MR angiography with midfemoral venous compression–initial experience. Radiology 2004; 230: 872–8.

24. Goyen M, Goehde SC, Herborn CU, Hunold P, Vogt FM, Gizewski ER, Lauenstein TC, Ajaj W, Forsting M, Debatin JF, Ruehm SG. MR-based full-body preventative cardiovascular and tumor imaging: technique and preliminary experience. Eur Radiol 2004; 14: 783–91.

25. Ruehm SG, Goyen M, Quick HH, Schleputz M, Schleputz H, Bosk S, Barkhausen J, Ladd ME, Debatin JF. [Whole-body MRA on a rolling table platform (AngioSURF)]. Rofo Fortschr Geb Rontgenstr Neuen Bildgeb Verfahr 2000; 172: 670–4.

26. Wachtell K, Ibsen H, Olsen MH, Laybourn C, Christoffersen JK, Norgaard H, Mantoni M, Lund JO. Prevalence of renal artery stenosis in patients with peripheral vascular disease and hypertension. J Hum Hypertens 1996; 10: 83–5.

27. Alexandrova NA, Gibson WC, Norris JW, Maggisano R. Carotid artery stenosis in peripheral vascular disease. J Vasc Surg 1996; 23: 645–9.

28. Marek J, Mills JL, Harvich J, Cui H, Fujitani RM. Utility of routine carotid duplex screening in patients who have claudication. J Vasc Surg 1996; 24: 572–7; discussion 577–9.

29. Goyen M, Ruehm SG, Barkhausen J, Kroger K, Ladd ME, Truemmler KH, Bosk S, Requardt M, Reykowski A, Debatin JF. Improved multi-station peripheral MR angiography with a dedicated vascular coil. J Magn Reson Imaging 2001; 13: 475–80.

30. Allardice JT, Allwright GJ, Wafula JM, Wyatt AP. High prevalence of abdominal aortic aneurysm in men with peripheral vascular disease: screening by ultrasonography. Br J Surg 1988; 75: 240–2.

31. Cooley DA, Carmichael MJ. Abdominal aortic aneurysm. Circulation. 1984; 70: I5–6.

32. Lederle FA, Walker JM, Reinke DB. Selective screening for abdominal aortic aneurysms with physical examination and ultrasound. Arch Intern Med 1988; 148: 1753–6.

33. Lederle FA, Johnson GR, Wilson SE, Chute EP, Littooy FN, Bandyk D, Krupski WC, Barone GW, Acher CW, Ballard DJ. Prevalence and associations of abdominal aortic aneurysm detected

through screening. Aneurysm Detection and Management (ADAM) Veterans Affairs Cooperative Study Group. Ann Intern Med 1997; 126: 441–9.

34. Lederle FA, Wilson SE, Johnson GR, Reinke DB, Littooy FN, Acher CW, Ballard DJ, Messina LM, Gordon IL, Chute EP, Krupski WC, Busuttil SJ, Barone GW, Sparks S, Graham LM, Rapp JH, Makaroun MS, Moneta GL, Cambria RA, Makhoul RG, Eton D, Ansel HJ, Freischlag JA, Bandyk D. Immediate repair compared with surveillance of small abdominal aortic aneurysms. N Engl J Med 2002; 346: 1437–44.

35. Coselli JS, Conklin LD, LeMaire SA. Thoracoabdominal aortic aneurysm repair: review and update of current strategies. Ann Thorac Surg 2002; 74: S1881–4; discussion S1892–8.

36. Coselli JS, LeMaire SA, Conklin LD, Koksoy C, Schmittling ZC. Morbidity and mortality after extent II thoracoabdominal aortic aneurysm repair. Ann Thorac Surg 2002; 73: 1107–15; discussion 1115–6.

37. Herborn CU, Vogt FM, Goyen M, Goehde SC, Ruehm SG, Forsting M. [Cardiovascular wholebody MRI: possibilities and limitations in prevention]. Radiologe 2004; 44: 826–34.

38. Goyen M, Lauenstein TC, Herborn CU, Debatin JF, Bosk S, Ruehm SG. 0.5 M Gd chelate (Magnevist) versus 1.0 M Gd chelate (Gadovist): dose-independent effect on image quality of pelvic three-dimensional MR-angiography. J Magn Reson Imaging 2001; 14: 602–7.

39. Goyen M, Herborn CU, Lauenstein TC, Barkhausen J, Veit P, Bosk S, Debatin J, Ruehm SG. Optimization of contrast dosage for gadobenate dimeglumine-enhanced high-resolution whole-body 3D magnetic resonance angiography. Invest Radiol 2002; 37: 263–8.

40. Goyen M, Herborn CU, Vogt FM, Kroger K, Verhagen R, Yang F, Bosk S, Debatin JF, Ruehm SG. Using a 1 M Gd-chelate (gadobutrol) for total-body three-dimensional MR angiography: preliminary experience. J Magn Reson Imaging 2003; 17: 565–71.

41. Herborn CU, Lauenstein TC, Ruehm SG, Bosk S, Debatin JF, Goyen M. Intraindividual comparison of gadopentetate dimeglumine, gadobenate dimeglumine, and gadobutrol for pelvic 3D magnetic resonance angiography. Invest Radiol 2003; 38: 27–33.

42. Knopp MV, Schoenberg SO, Rehm C, Floemer F, von Tengg-Kobligk H, Bock M, Hentrich HR. Assessment of gadobenate dimeglumine for magnetic resonance angiography: phase I studies. Invest Radiol 2002; 37: 706–15.

43. Knopp MV, Giesel FL, von Tengg-Kobligk H, Radeleff J, Requardt M, Kirchin MA, Hentrich HR. Contrast-enhanced MR angiography of the run-off vasculature: intraindividual comparison of gadobenate dimeglumine with gadopentetate dimeglumine. J Magn Reson Imaging 2003; 17: 694–702.

44. Kroencke TJ, Wasser MN, Pattynama PM, Barentsz JO, Grabbe E, Marchal G, Knopp MV, Schneider G, Bonomo L, Pennell DJ, del Maschio A, Hentrich HR, Dapra M, Kirchin MA, Spinazzi A, Taupitz M, Hamm B. Gadobenate dimeglumine-enhanced MR angiography of the abdominal aorta and renal arteries. AJR Am J Roentgenol 2002; 179: 1573–82.

45. Wikstrom J, Wasser MN, Pattynama PM, Bonomo L, Hamm B, Del Maschio A, Knopp MV, Marchal G, Barentsz JO, Oudkerk M, Hentrich HR, Dapra M, Kirchin MA, Shen N, Spinazzi A, Ahlstrom H. Gadobenate dimeglumine-enhanced magnetic resonance angiography of the pelvic arteries. Invest Radiol 2003; 38: 504–15.

46. Lauffer RB, Parmelee DJ, Ouellet HS, Dolan RP, Sajiki H, Scott DM, Bernard PJ, Buchanan EM, Ong KY, Tyeklar Z, Midelfort KS, McMurry TJ, Walovitch RC. MS-325: a small-molecule vascular imaging agent for magnetic resonance imaging. Acad Radiol 1996; 3 Suppl 2: S356–8.

47. Lauffer RB, Parmelee DJ, Dunham SU, Ouellet HS, Dolan RP, Witte S, McMurry TJ, Walovitch RC. MS-325: albumin-targeted contrast agent for MR angiography. Radiology 1998; 207: 529–38.

48. Kim WY, Danias PG, Stuber M, Flamm SD, Plein S, Nagel E, Langerak SE, Weber OM, Pedersen EM, Schmidt M, Botnar RM, Manning WJ. Coronary magnetic resonance angiography for the detection of coronary stenoses. N Engl J Med 2001; 345: 1863–9.

49. Manning WJ, Stuber M, Danias PG, Botnar RM, Yeon SB, Aepfelbacher FC. Coronary magnetic resonance imaging: current status. Curr Probl Cardiol 2002; 27: 275–333.

4 Whole-body MR angiography using the intravascular contrast agent Vasovist®

Konstantin Nikolaou

4.1 Introduction

A number of studies have investigated the feasibility of "whole-body" MRA [1, 2], meaning anatomic coverage of most, but hardly all, vascular territories of the body. In order to assess vascular pathologies in more than one vascular region, several of these studies utilized dedicated rolling platforms that are combined with fast imaging in order to cover the entire body within a short scan time [3]. First results have been promising, but come along with a somewhat reduced spatial resolution due to the necessity of fast imaging and coverage of a large field of view (FOV). In subsequent studies on multi-station MRA implemented on new MR imagers with matrix coils and applying parallel imaging techniques, coverage of the whole vasculature without the need of re-positioning the patient has been demonstrated on standard scanner hardware [4]. Still, all studies described limitations and compromises in either spatial resolution or anatomic coverage due to the limited time-frame during first-pass of the contrast agent. Several approaches have been tested to extend the duration of arterial phase imaging, such as the use of venous compression (VENCO) for imaging the peripheral run-off [5, 6].

In addition to these continuing improvements in software (i.e. MR sequences and acquisition strategies) and hardware (e.g., dedicated 32-channel whole-body MRI scanner), the development of new and refined MR contrast agents will further improve and change imaging strategies in whole-body MRA. With the introduction of intravascular paramagnetic contrast agents known as blood pool agents for enhancing MR angiographic images, limitations of today's whole-body MRA might be overcome, and imaging strategies in multi-station MRA could further be developed and improved [7]. One such intravascular compound is Vasovist® (Gadofosveset, MS-325, Schering, Berlin, Germany). This compound is a small-molecule contrast agent that binds noncovalently to serum albumin. This reversible albumin binding of Vasovist® enhances the paramagnetic effectiveness of gadolinium and allows lower contrast agent doses than are needed with conventional MR agents [8]. Most of all, the albumin-binding characteristic extends the vascular lifetime of the agent, and thus allows longer vascular imaging time, potentially higher spatial resolution, and larger anatomic coverage. During the equilibrium or "steady-state" phase of the contrast, several portions of the body vasculature can be examined consecutively without additional injections of contrast required. Thus, by combining new 32-channel MR systems with matrix coils and intravascular contrast agents, whole-body MRA can be performed with only a single injection of contrast, scanning the complete vasculature without compromises in spatial resolution or anatomic coverage, and without repositioning the patient.

4.2 Whole body MRA implementing Vasovist® – technical aspects

The latest MR acquisition techniques using conventional, extracellular contrast agents can readily achieve a sufficient and optimized SNR that supports the spatial, sub-millimeter resolution required for detailed analysis of small branch arteries. However, time constraints induced by the short intra-arterial presence of any extracellular contrast agent limit data acquisition times and hence do not permit full exploitation of the spatial resolution potential. With the introduction of blood pool contrast agents, this paradigm could be shifted [7]. The strongly albumin-binding gadolinium chelate Gadofosveset has a half-life time of about 15 hours. Initial experience shows that Gadofosveset could allow for imaging of more than 1 hour while maintaining a sufficiently high signal-to-noise ratio (SNR) during steady-state imaging. The contrast can be injected with a low flow rate of 1 ml/s. Gadofosveset is a gadolinium-based small-molecule (molecular weight, 975.88) contrast agent designed specifically for MR angiography. Gadofosveset is 80%–96% noncovalently bound to albumin in human plasma and is primarily excreted renally. In plasma, Gadofosveset exhibits a relaxivity at 1.5 T that is approximately 5 to 7 times that of Gd-DTPA [8, 9].

Administration volume of Vasovist® is calculated according to the following formula:

$$[Subject\ weight\ (kg) \times 0.03\ mmol/kg]/[0.25\ mmol/mL]$$

For example, in a patient with a body weight of about 75 kg, the total injection volume would be 9 ml. Applying an injection flow rate of 1 ml/s, this results in an injection duration of 9 seconds.

After injection of an intravascular contrast agent such as Vasovist®, two acquisition phases can be discerned. During the arterial first-pass, or dynamic phase, typical arterial angiograms can be obtained, similar to any arterial angiogram acquired with conventional extracellular MR contrast agents. In this dynamic phase after contrast injection, angiograms of a single vascular bed, e.g. the carotid arteries, renal arteries, or peripheral arteries can typically be obtained. Alternatively, time-resolved imaging could be performed during the first pass of the contrast, e.g. perfusion imaging of the lung or kidney. With implementation of a new 32-channel whole-body 1.5 T MRI scanner with matrix coils and parallel imaging (Magnetom Avanto, Siemens Medical Solutions, Erlangen, Germany), it is even possible to scan two vessel territories during the first pass of the intravascular contrast compound: E.g., the carotid arteries and lower leg arteries can be acquired after a single contrast injection, since with this 32-channel MR imager, table movement is faster than the passage of the contrast bolus, and purely arterial angiograms of the lower legs can be acquired after imaging the carotid arteries. Figure 4.1 shows the subsequent filling of calf arteries and veins after a single injection of contrast during repeated first-pass imaging of Vasovist®. The acquisition time is 29 seconds per phase, and spatial resolution is 1.0×1.0×1.0 mm.

Following this dynamic phase, the contrast compound distributes in the complete body vasculature, both arterial and venous system, and reaches an equilibrium phase after about 5 minutes. In this steady-state, or equilibrium phase, very high spatial resolutions can be achieved, as certain vascular beds not affected by cardiac or respiratory motion, such as the lower extremities, can be scanned for several minutes. Table 4.1 gives typical imaging parameters for first-pass and steady-state imaging of various vessel territories. In a Phase II study

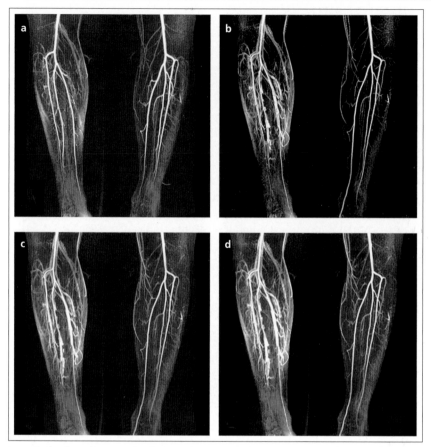

Figure 4.1a–d The four data sets **(a–d)** show the subsequent successive filling of calf arteries and veins during the first pass of Vasovist®, displayed as subtracted maximum-intensity projections (MIP). Data from a healthy volunteer (injection rate = 1.0 ml/s, TR/TE= 4.3/1.4 ms, FA = 30°, resolutions = 1.0×1.0×1.0 mm3; 29 s acquisition time per phase).

performing multi-station MRA with Vasovist®, a spatial resolution of up to 0.074 mm³ (i.e., 0.42 mm isotropic voxel length) was realized during the steady-state phase, within an acquisition time of about 6 minutes [10].

4.3 Whole-body MRA implementing Vasovist® – potential in clinical application

High-resolution, multi-station MRA is a fairly new diagnostic approach to detect multiple manifestations of systemic atherosclerosis. Using standard MR sequences, imagers, and protocols, the diagnostic accuracy of MRA as compared to catheter-based angiography may still be limited, even when performing MR angiography of single vascular beds. For example, in a recent multi-center trial comparing renal MRA and X-ray angiography, the combined sensitivity and specificity was as low as 64% and 92%, respectively [11]. Recent publications have shown that by using optimized acquisition techniques like parallel imaging or high-field scanners, the spatial resolution required for a reliable diagnosis of significant renal artery stenoses can be achieved [12]. With the implementation of these parallel imaging techniques, multi-station MRA benefits from an increase in spatial or temporal resolution at low cost in scan time [13]. Recently, it could be shown that by integrating parallel imaging techniques into a comprehensive whole-body cardiovascular screening protocol on a 32-channel MR imager, all relevant vascular systems can be examined without compromising spatial or temporal resolution [4]. Still, all these techniques share two limitations:

1) MR angiograms can only be acquired during the relatively short period of the arterial contrast passage, and
2) Several contrast injections are needed to cover the complete body vasculature.

Here, application of an intravascular contrast agent such as Vasovist® could result in extended imaging time, potentially higher spatial resolution, and larger anatomic coverage. Below, initial experiences of a Phase II study combining state-of-the-art MRI techniques with Vasovist® are reported using a setup as described above (combining Vasovist® and a 32-channel MR imager with parallel imaging techniques for high-resolution, multi-station MRA, Table 4.1) [10]. In this study, 10 healthy volunteers and 10 patients with proven atherosclerotic disease underwent whole-body MRA. In the patients, results of whole-body Vasovist®-enhanced MR angiograms were compared to state-of-the-art MRA protocols using conventional Gd-chelates as the reference standard.

Results of this preliminary study are indeed encouraging. In the dynamic phase or first pass of Vasovist®, MR angiograms of both the carotid and the lower leg arteries with pure arterial contrast were consistently obtained without venous overlay. For this first-pass imaging, typical MRA protocol parameters as used for extracellular contrast agents were applied, as acquisition strategies during first-pass are very similar to conventional arterial MR angiograms. Due to the higher relaxivity of Vasovist® as compared to conventional MR contrast agents, a low flow rate of 1 ml/s and a total contrast volume of about 7–10 ml were sufficient for a very high arterial signal. As the relaxivity of Vasovist® is 5–7 times higher than for conventional, 0.5 molar extracellular contrast agent (at 1.5 T), and since it is being

Table 4.1 Whole-body MRA using Vasovist®: First-pass vs. steady-state imaging with spatial resolution and acquisition time

First-Pass Imaging		
Vascular Territory	**Spatial Resolution**	**Acquisition Time**
Carotid Arteries	$1.0 \times 1.0 \times 1.0$ mm = **1.0 mm³**	0:12 min
Lower Leg	$1.0 \times 1.0 \times 1.0$ mm = **1.0 mm³**	0:29 min
Steady-State Imaging		
Carotid Arteries	$0.8 \times 0.8 \times 0.8$ mm = **0.512 mm³**	0:40 min
Thorax	$1.0 \times 1.0 \times 1.0$ mm = **1.0 mm³**	0:37 min
Abdomen	$1.0 \times 1.0 \times 1.0$ mm = **1.0 mm³**	0:35 min
Upper Leg	$0.5 \times 0.5 \times 0.5$ mm = **0.125 mm³**	5:46 min
Knee	$0.5 \times 0.5 \times 0.5$ mm = **0.125 mm³**	3:40 min
Lower Leg	$0.42 \times 0.42 \times 0.42$ mm = **0.074 mm³**	6:16 min

injected at 1 ml/s, this would translate into an injection rate of about 5–7 ml/s using conventional contrast agent. This might be one reason for the very high vascular signal and high image quality of the Vasovist® first-pass data. Potentially, this benefit of a high SNR during the first pass of Vasovist® could also be advantageous for time-resolved imaging, potentially enabling assessment of absolute parenchymal organ perfusion.

During steady-state imaging of Vasovist®-enhanced MRA, acquisition strategies have to be adapted and changed significantly. Due to the long half-life time of the contrast, steady-state imaging can be performed for up to several minutes in one vascular bed. Thus, especially in vascular territories not affected by cardiac or respiratory motion, very high spatial resolutions below 0.10 mm^3 can be achieved (e.g., in the lower leg). As compared to conventional first-pass MRA techniques, performed at about 1.0 mm^3 spatial resolution, this means an increase in spatial resolution by a factor of 10, comparing voxel sizes. However, as the matrix size used can be as high as 1024×1024 in certain vascular beds, long acquisition times of several minutes can occur. Also, image reconstruction time increases with these high matrices, up to a maximum of about 10 minutes reconstruction time for 128 images at a matrix of 1024×1024, which has to be noted as a drawback of the technique, as an exam has to be both accurate and patient/interpreter friendly, maintaining a high patient throughput. Still, despite the long acquisition times at 0.125 mm^3 and 0.074 mm^3 spatial resolutions, image quality was rated as "excellent" in almost all cases of the study described above. In the patient group, however, in a few cases image quality of the high resolution lower leg data sets was diminished due to movement artifacts. Obviously, the risk of movement artifacts possibly impairing image quality directly increases with mounting acquisition times. On the other hand, especially in the lower leg, where small-caliber arterial and venous vascular structures are in close vicinity, only at a high spatial resolution of 0.5 or 0.42 mm voxel length can the arterial and venous vessels be clearly differentiated (Fig. 4.2). In data sets with spatial resolution of 0.8 and 1.0 mm voxel length, venous over-

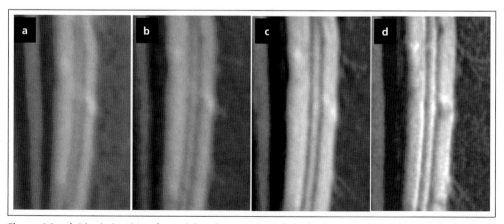

Figure 4.2a–d Discrimination of arterial and venous vessels in the lower leg. In this example from a 30- year-old healthy volunteer, magnified views of the anterior tibial artery (vessel in the center), accompanied by two veins (vessels to the left and right), are displayed, with increasing spatial resolutions (**a–d**, isotropic voxel lengths: 1.0 mm^3, 0.,512 mm^3, 0.125 mm^3, 0.075 mm^3). With increasing spatial resolution, the central arterial vessel is delineated more and more clearly, proving demonstrating the dependency of arterial versus venous vessel delineation from on spatial resolution in the steady-state phase images.

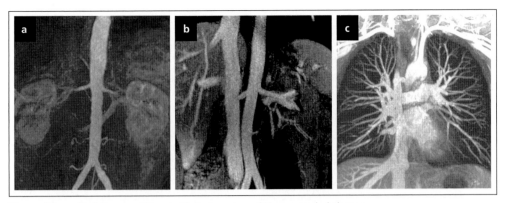

Figure 4.3a–c First-Pass and Steady-State Imaging of thorax and abdomen:
a) First-Pass Imaging: During arterial first-pass of Vasovist®, pure arterial phase images of the renal arteries can be obtained after a single injection of contrast, with an isotropic spatial resolution of 1.0 mm³, acquired during an 18 s breath-hold. Only minor vessel wall irregularities of the aortic wall can be seen, no significant stenoses.
b, c) Steady-State Imaging: Maximum-intensity projections (MIP) of 20 mm thickness of the thorax and abdomen. During steady-state imaging of the thorax and abdomen, a spatial resolution of 1.0 mm³ isotropic voxel size was acquired in a 32 s and 30 s breath-hold, respectively. Both arterial and venous structures are homogeneously enhanced, maintaining a sufficiently high signal-to-noise ratio (SNR) for diagnostic purposes. No significant disease was found in this patient.

lay is still present and can result in a potential diagnostic problem. As a compromise, a spatial resolution of 0.5 mm voxel length seems to be acceptable for imaging the peripheral run-off, enabling a clear differentiation of arterial and venous structures during the equilibrium phase of the contrast material and maintaining an acceptable acquisition time of 3 to 5 minutes for the thigh, knee, and calf level.

In other vascular territories acquired during steady-state of Vasovist®, cardiac and breathing motion artifacts can cause considerable problems concerning acquisition optimization. For example, in the thorax and abdomen, acquisition time is limited to the time frame of a single breath-hold; thus, the potential of the intravascular contrast for high spatial resolution, requiring acquisition times of several minutes, can not fully be exploited. Refined acquisition techniques using free-breathing navigators, possibly combined with ECG-gating, could be effective for both the thoracic and abdominal vasculature for overcoming these hurdles. Still, even during the relatively short period of a breath-hold, SNR of the Gadofosveset data during steady-state is high enough to enable acquisition of fully diagnostic MRA data sets (Fig. 4.3).

Concerning the diagnostic accuracy reported in the Phase II trial, Vasovist®-enhanced MRA data sets yielded the full diagnostic information as compared to the reference imaging modalities, showing a high sensitivity for significant vascular diseases at the carotid arteries or the lower leg arteries. In general, first-pass and steady-state images can be read in a combined fashion, providing complementary information (Figs. 4.4 and 4.5). Combining this information could be performed as follows: For a first overview, the first-pass MIP data are very helpful, similar to conventional first-pass MRA data sets using extracellular contrast agents. In a second step, source images of both the first-pass and steady-state data should be read, possibly with additional three-dimensional reformations, e.g. multiplanar

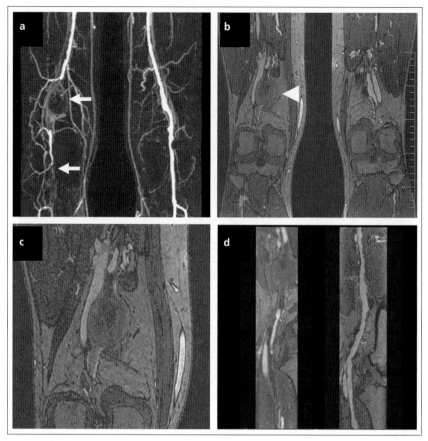

Figure 4.4a–d 54-year-old male patient with a long history of diabetes, suffering from increasing claudication in his right leg. The subtracted maximum-intensity projection of the first-pass data of Vasovist®-enhanced MRA shows significant disease, with an occlusion of the right superficial femoral artery and right popliteal artery (**a**, arrows). The coronal steady-state Vasovist®-enhanced images of the thigh and knee with a spatial resolution of 0.5 mm isotropic voxel length (0.125 mm³) show a large aneurysm of the right distal superficial femoral artery (SFA), with a thrombotic occlusion of the vessel, substituted by collateral vessels (**b**, arrowhead, **c**, magnified view). Performing curved multiplanar reformations (MPR), the course of the distal SFA and popliteal artery can be displayed for the right and the left leg, showing the sites of vessel occlusions of the right leg **(d)**, as well as all details on vessel wall irregularities on the left side.

reformations (MPR). However, it has to be admitted that some special reconstruction techniques, such as three-dimensional Volume Rendering (VRT), which have been described as being helpful in the comprehensive assessment of MRA data sets [14], can not be used with the steady-state data due to venous overlay. Earlier Phase III study results on the use of Vasovist® in peripheral arterial disease had already shown significant improvement in effectiveness over non-contrast-enhanced MRA at a dose of 0.03 mmol/kg, and a safe and effective MR evaluation of patients with aortoiliac occlusive disease [15, 16]. However, these studies were limited to a single vessel territory and compared diagnostic accuracy to non-enhanced MR angiographic techniques.

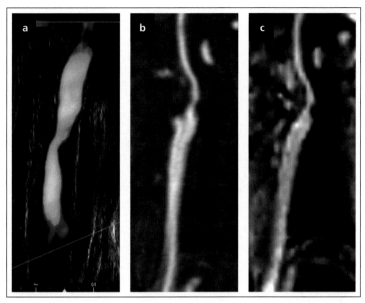

Figure 4.5a–c 65-year-old male patient, suffering from transient ischemic attacks. The reference imaging modality, i.e. color-coded Doppler ultrasound, showed a 75% stenosis with a maximal flow velocity of 1.7 m/s **(a)**. The maximum-intensity projection (MIP) of the first-pass Vasovist®-enhanced data (spatial resolution, 1 mm³) shows a significant stenosis in the proximal right internal carotid artery **(b)**. A multiplanar reformation (MPR) of the steady-state images at 0.8 mm isotropic resolution demonstrates the diagnostic value of both the first-pass and steady-state data, confirming the ICA stenosis **(c)**.

4.4   Conclusions and future perspectives

Up to now, long acquisition times and restrictions in temporal and spatial resolution were limiting factors for using MRI as a tool for multi-station or "whole-body" angiography. By combining intravascular contrast agents such as Vasovist®, new acquisition techniques such as parallel imaging and multislice sequences, and newly developed hardware such as a 32-channel MRI imager, these problems might be overcome. After careful optimization and adaptation of sequence parameters, multi-station MRA using an intravascular contrast agent can be performed with high spatial resolution, maintaining a high diagnostic accuracy. First-pass imaging is feasible and delivers purely arterial angiograms comparable to state-of-the-art first-pass angiograms of any given vascular bed using standard, extracellular contrast agents. During steady-state, very high spatial resolutions can be achieved that have not been reported for three-dimensional MR angiograms so far. Future work will have to deal with optimization of scan time, reconstruction time, and image interpretation strategies of steady-state data, as well as further optimization of the image quality during steady-state imaging, especially in the thorax and abdomen.

Bibliography

1. Ruehm SG, Goyen M, Barkhausen J, Kroger K, Bosk S, Ladd ME, Debatin JF. Rapid magnetic resonance angiography for detection of atherosclerosis. Lancet 2001; 357: 1086–91.

2. Herborn CU, Goyen M, Quick HH, Bosk S, Massing S, Kroeger K, Stoesser D, Ruehm SG, Debatin JF. Whole-body 3D MR angiography of patients with peripheral arterial occlusive disease. AJR Am J Roentgenol 2004; 182: 1427–1434.

3. Ruehm SG, Goyen M, Quick HH, Schleputz M, Schleputz H, Bosk S, Barkhausen J, Ladd ME, Debatin JF. [Whole-body MRA on a rolling table platform (AngioSURF)]. Rofo 2000; 172: 670–674.

4. Kramer H, Schoenberg SO, Nikolaou K, Huber A, Struwe A, Winnik E, Wintersperger BJ, Dietrich O, Kiefer B, Reiser MF. Cardiovascular screening with parallel imaging techniques and a whole-body MR imager. Radiology 2005; 236: 300–310.

5. Vogt FM, Ajaj W, Hunold P, Herborn CU, Quick HH, Debatin JF, Ruehm SG. Venous compression at high-spatial-resolution three-dimensional MR angiography of peripheral arteries. Radiology 2004; 233: 913–920.

6. Bilecen D, Jager KA, Aschwanden M, Heidecker HG, Schulte AC, Bongartz G. Cuff-compression of the proximal calf to reduce venous contamination in contrast-enhanced stepping-table magnetic Resonance angiography. Acta Radiol 2004; 45: 510–515.

7. Perrault LP, Edelman RR, Baum RA, Yucel EK, Weisskoff RM, Shamsi K, Mohler ER. MR angiography with gadofosveset trisodium for peripheral vascular disease: phase II trial. Radiology 2003; 229: 811–820.

8. Lauffer RB, Parmelee DJ, Dunham SU, Ouellet HS, Dolan RP, Witte S, McMurry TJ, Walovitch RC. MS-325: albumin-targeted contrast agent for MR angiography. Radiology 1998; 207: 529–38.

9. Rohrer M, Bauer H, Mintorovitch J, Requardt M, Weinmann HJ. Comparison of magnetic properties of MRI contrast media solutions at different magnetic field strengths. Invest Radiol 2005; 40: 715–724.

10. Nikolaou K, Kramer H, Grosse C, Clevert D, Dietrich O, Hartmann M, Chamberlin P, Assmann S, Reiser MF, Schoenberg SO. High spatial resolution multi-station MRA using parallel imaging and a blood pool contrast agent: Initial experience. Radiology 2006; in press.

11. Vasbinder GB, Nelemans PJ, Kessels AG, Kroon AA, Maki JH, Leiner T, Beek FJ, Korst MB, Flobbe K, de Haan MW, van Zwam WH, Postma CT, Hunink MG, de Leeuw PW, van Engelshoven JM. Accuracy of computed tomographic angiography and magnetic resonance angiography for diagnosing renal artery stenosis. Ann Intern Med 2004; 141: 674–682.

12. Michaely HJ, Nael K, Schoenberg SO, Finn JP, Laub G, Reiser MF, Ruehm SG. The feasibility of spatial high-resolution magnetic resonance angiography (MRA) of the renal arteries at 3.0 T. Rofo 2005; 177: 800–804.

13. Weiger M, Pruessmann KP, Kassner A, Roditi G, Lawton T, Reid A, Boesiger P. Contrast-enhanced 3D MRA using SENSE. J Magn Reson Imaging 2000; 12: 671–677.

14. Mallouhi A, Schocke M, Judmaier W, Wolf C, Dessl A, Czermak BV, Waldenberger P, Jaschke WR. 3D MR angiography of renal arteries: comparison of volume rendering and maximum intensity projection algorithms. Radiology 2002; 223: 509–516.

15. Goyen M, Edelman M, Perreault P, O'Riordan E, Bertoni H, Taylor J, Siragusa D, Sharafuddin M, Mohler ER, III, Breger R, Yucel EK, Shamsi K, Weisskoff RM. MR angiography of aortoiliac occlusive disease: a phase III study of the safety and effectiveness of the blood-pool contrast agent MS-325. Radiology 2005; 236: 825–833.

16. Rapp JH, Wolff SD, Quinn SF, Soto JA, Meranze SG, Muluk S, Blebea J, Johnson SP, Rofsky NM, Duerinckx A, Foster GS, Kent KC, Moneta G, Middlebrook MR, Narra VR, Toombs BD, Pollak J, Yucel EK, Shamsi K, Weisskoff RM. Aortoiliac occlusive disease in patients with known or suspected peripheral vascular disease: safety and efficacy of gadofosveset-enhanced MR angiography – multicenter comparative phase III study. Radiology 2005; 236: 71–78.

5 Whole-body MRI for the diagnosis of musculoskeletal diseases

Sabine Lenk

5.1 Introduction

The previous imaging methods used in whole-body diagnostics of the locomotive system – conventional X-ray, scintigraphy and positron emission tomography (PET) – show limited specificity and anatomical depictability, as well as entailing radiation exposure. MRI has already become established in the musculoskeletal diagnostics of various anatomical regions, especially in the spinal cord and joints.

The introduction of the whole-body MRI technique opens up new possibilities for the diagnosis of diseases of the locomotive system. Especially in cases of chronic polyarthritis, systemic inflammatory connective tissue diseases, and musculoskeletal development disorders, whole-body MRI facilitates depiction of the pattern of occurrence and provides assistance in locating the optimal region for biopsy as part of initial diagnostics of the related disease. Whole-body MRI is also outstandingly suitable in tracking the progress of these diseases (therapy success/advances of the disease/potential transformation etc.) while avoiding examination techniques involving radiation exposure with frequently young patients.

Important diagnostic options especially arise for whole-body MRI in polymyositis, muscular dystrophy, fibromatoses, multiple cartilaginous exostoses, polyostotic dysplasia, vasculitis, rheumatoid arthritis and ankylosing spondylitis. For diagnostics of the joints, it should be mentioned as a restriction that high-resolution, one-stop imaging including the small joints of the hand and foot is not possible with whole-body MRI. In the case of an indication in these areas – e.g. rheumatoid arthritis – a dedicated surface coil should be used.

Whole-body MRI offers a very sensitive method for staging and for the control of therapy in bone metastases in identified primary tumors, lymphoma infiltration of the skeleton, plasmacytomas and polyostotic tumors. Whole-body MRI is only of limited suitability with low specificity for primary diagnostics of bone tumors.

For whole-body MRI indications, it should be borne in mind that the use of coronal TIRM overview sequences alone is not sufficient for an adequate musculoskeletal diagnosis and therefore further specific sequences are required. The examination protocol must be matched to the respective disease, whereby the examination times at a field strength of 1.5 Tesla extend to a total of approx. 45–60 minutes. Reductions in measurement times are to be expected with the introduction of 3.0 Tesla whole-body MRI systems currently undergoing validation.

This chapter provides an overview of the possibilities and limitations of whole-body MRI in the diagnosis of diseases of the musculoskeletal system. An efficient examination protocol for whole-body musculoskeletal diagnosis is proposed, which takes account of current technical advancements.

5.2 Imaging diagnostics

5.2.1 Conventional MRI

Besides the absence of radiation exposure, the advantages of magnetic resonance imaging over other imaging techniques lie in the high resolution of anatomical detail, the good presentation of bone and soft tissue structures, as well as its high sensitivity and specificity towards pathological changes. MRI has become well established over many years in the specific examination of joint, muscle, and bone lesions of individual regions of the body. However, due to technical limitations, the use of MRI for routine whole-body diagnostics is still only possible to a limited extent. The reason is firstly the reduced spatial resolution in the use of the whole-body coil and secondly, the time-consuming and impractical replacement of coils for use as surface coils.

5.2.2 Whole-body MRI

With the introduction of the table movement technique and use of whole-body coils or a phased array coil (Angio*SURF* technique, see Chap. 1), whole-body MRI examination became feasible for routine use. Since 2004, 1.5 Tesla MRI systems (Avanto, Siemens Medical

Table 5.1 Sequence protocol for whole-body musculoskeletal MRI at 1.5 Tesla

Sequence	Orientation	TR (ms)	TE (ms)	TI (ms)	FOV	Resolution	Section thickness (mm)	Acquisition time (min)
TIRM whole-body (5×)	coronal	5800–9760	87	150	480	1.8 × 1.3 × 5.0	5	11:13
TIRM neck	axial	6180	59	150	220	1.2 × 0.9 × 5.0	5	2:17
TIRM thorax	axial	4480	100	150	380	1.8 × 1.2 × 6.0	6	0:48
TIRM abdomen	axial	4480	100	150	380	1.8 × 1.2 × 6.0	6	0:48
TIRM pelvis	axial	7100	70	150	360	1.3 × 1.0 × 5.0	5	4:31
TIRM thigh	axial	6150	70	150	330	1.5 × 1.2 × 5.0	5	3:31
TIRM lower leg	axial	6150	70	150	330	1.5 × 1.2 × 5.0	5	3:31
T1 SE whole-body (5×)	coronal	400–577	11	n	480	1.6 × 1.3 × 5.0	5	15:10
T1 SE whole spine	sagittal	476	11	n	400	1.4 × 1.0 × 3.0	4	1:38
T2 TSE whole spine	sagittal	3360	100	n	400	1.4 × 1.0 × 3.0	4	2:39
T1 SE fatsat post i.v. CA where applicable	specifically for pathological result							

Systems, Erlangen, Germany) equipped with a whole-body coil system (76 coil elements) and 32 radiofrequency channels have been available, with which a coronal TIRM whole-body overview can be obtained at high spatial resolution with a 205 cm field of view within approx. 14 min. A targeted examination of individual regions of the body can then be undertaken dependent on the clinical issues to be addressed without further repositioning. The common spin-echo and gradient-echo sequences are available for this purpose.

For musculoskeletal whole-body MRI diagnostics, coronal and axial T1w spin-echo and axial TIRM sequences are available for basic diagnostics in addition to coronal TIRM over-

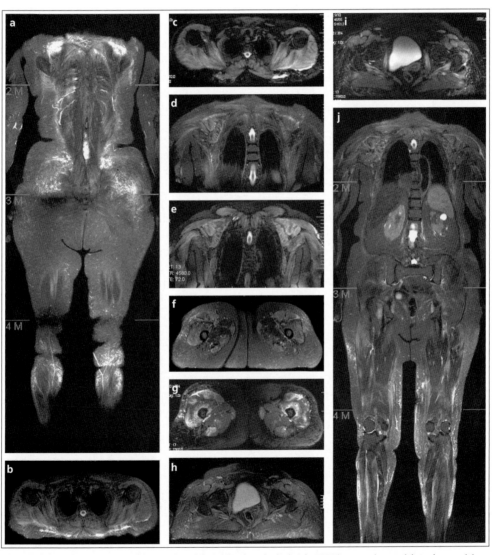

Figure 5.1a–j Comparison of 1.5 Tesla with 3.0 Tesla whole-body MRI in a patient with polymyositis. Diffuse infiltration of polymyositis in almost all muscle groups of the trunk and extremities.
(a, j) Coronal TIRM overview; **(b, d, f, h)** 1.5 Tesla – axial and coronal TIRM; **(c, e, g, i)** 3.0 Tesla – axial and coronal TIRM.

view sequences. Sagittal T1w-SE and T2w-TSE sequences are also acquired to examine the whole spine. Dependent on the problem, axial and coronal T1w-SE sequences with the fat suppression (FS) technique following administration of an intravenous contrast agent (0.2 mmol Gd-DTPA/kg body weight) can be specifically performed. Intravenous contrast agent administration has been shown to be effective, especially as part of whole-body tumor staging while searching for soft tissue and bone metastases, but also in the investigation of inflammatory muscle and joint conditions.

For the large joints, both a primary musculoskeletal overview screening and a directed high-resolution examination are possible in a single examination session. Problems arise in the attempt to simultaneously image the small joints (hands, elbow joint, feet) with high resolution. Here the whole-body coil system succeeds, at least for a rough diagnostic representation. The unfavorable placement of the hands beside the body or on the thighs rather above the head is also problematic. Therefore, if there is a need for detailed diagnostics of the small joints, a separate examination using selective surface coils should be supplemented.

Difficulties sometimes arise with patients with a stout physique in the full depiction of the shoulder joint, which in such cases may be located on the margins of the maximum field of view.

The following proposed sequence protocol can be used to perform comprehensive musculoskeletal whole-body diagnostics within a reasonable period of 45 min. As required, a specific examination of pathological findings using T1w-SE-FS sequences can be supplemented following the administration of an intravenous contrast agent. A broad spectrum of clinical investigations, such as multifocal inflammations, tumors or degenerative changes of the bones, joints and muscular system, as well as musculoskeletal development disorders can be covered with this protocol (Table 5.1).

Currently, 3.0 Tesla whole-body MRI systems are undergoing clinical testing, and the initial results look promising, especially in regard to a reduction in measurement time. A significant time savings with unchanged image quality is expected following the introduction of new high-field technology, at least for some indications (Fig. 5.1).

5.3 Clinical symptoms

The clinical symptoms of the musculoskeletal group of diseases, for which whole-body MRI appears effective, are presented in the following section.

5.3.1 Bones

5.3.1.1 Polytrauma

In a study from 2003 [4], Green et al. carried out an MRI examination of the full spine with 127 polytraumatized patients and in 77% of the cases detected an additional vertebral injury in a secondary accident level which was not see on conventional X-ray examinations. Sagittal fat-saturated T2w-TSE sequences, as well as sagittal and axial T1w-SE sequences, were employed. This study presents an interesting approach for using whole-body MRI following moderate polytrauma (e.g. minor traffic accidents where an expert opinion for insurance purposes must be formulated) in the detection of multi-station injuries of the skeletal system not seen on plain films. However, for a routine examination of the acutely traumatized patient, CT is still to be preferred as a faster method with better monitoring options.

An important indication for whole-body MRI is given in the case of battered child syndrome (child abuse). The use of a coronal whole-body STIR overview sequence with subsequent specific examination of the affected body regions is recommended, especially in comparison with bone scintigraphy.

5.3.1.2 Tumors and metastases

Whole-body MRI has advantages for staging and progress monitoring of multifocal tumors and bone metastases.

Bone metastases are the third most common manifestation of distant metastasis of malignant tumors and the most frequently occurring bone tumor. 80% of bone metastases originate from a breast, prostate, bronchial, thyroid or renal carcinoma. Only 10% of bone metastases appear primarily [15]. There are already several publications on the significance of whole-body MRI with the automated stepping movement technique for skeletal metastasis [1, 5, 9, 10, 13, 16]. In a study conducted by Tausig et al. in 2000 [10] in 20 patients with bone metastasis from a breast carcinoma, MRI in the regions of the thorax and skull was considered as an inferior method compared with scintigraphy on account of artifacts, although only STIR sequences were used. On the other hand, a study from Engelhardt et al. from 2004 [1] showed MRI (sensitivity 92%, specificity 90%, detection accuracy 91%) to be superior to scintigraphy (83%, 80%, 82%, respectively) in the diagnosis of bone metastases in 22 female patients with breast carcinoma. Coronal STIR sequences, axial T2w-TSE sequences, and, for the spine, sagittal T1w-SE sequences were used. Reference was made to the high potential of whole-body MRI for screening of bone metastases; however, scintigraphy was still preferred as the cheaper method for routine use.

A study from 2000 conducted by Steinborn et al. [16] with 18 patients with bone metastases from different primary tumors compared whole-body MRI (sensitivity 91.4%) with bone scintigraphy (84.8%) and indicates the advantage of MRI, especially in the assessment of complications with spinal metastasis. T1w-SE, STIR, and T2w-TSE-FS sequences were used. Lauenstein et al. found a good correlation between whole-body MRI and bone scintigraphy in a study from 2002 [13] as part of a tumor staging protocol for 8 patients with bone metastasis, even though only 3D T1w-GE-FS sequences were used following administration of an intravenous contrast agent (see Chap. 7). In an article from 2005 [5], Daldrup-Link et al. refer to difficulties in MRI in bone barrow assessment in children and preferred the use of axial T1w-SE sequences in the detection of bone metastases. In this work, MRI (sensitivity 82%), FDG-PET (90%) and bone scintigraphy (71%) were compared for children with bone metastases from different tumors. While PET was superior, weaknesses of MRI were mainly found in the diagnosis in the region of the small peripheral bones and the ribs.

The use of very sensitive whole-body TIRM sequences alone is not sufficient for specific bone marrow diagnostics. Supplementary T1w-SE and T2w-TSE sequences are required especially in the spinal column. Irrespective of the MRI technique, the differentiation between residual hematopoietic bone marrow and neoplastic bone marrow infiltration still causes problems. Besides considering the age-specific distribution pattern of the red and yellow bone marrow and the underlying disease of the patient, the use of in-phase and out-of-phase pulse sequences is recommended by some authors [5, 16]. The administration of intravenous contrast agent has not been shown to be helpful in most cases for differentiating bone marrow lesions.

Given the very diverse study results in the literature so far, larger scale clinical studies with unified study designs, selected according to tumor entities and large populations, are required to verify the significance of whole-body MRI in the diagnosis of bone metastases in comparison with other imaging methods (Fig. 5.2.)

5.3.1.3 Plasmacytoma

Plasmacytomas are monoclonal B-lymphocyte tumors with increased immunoglobin synthesis and infiltration of the red bone marrow. Given a variable osteolytic pattern of occurrence in the skeletal system (solitary, multiple, diffuse, disseminated), there is a higher incidence in the skull, the spinal column, the ribs, the pelvis and the femur. MRI using fat suppressed T2w sequences (TIRM/T2w-TSE-FS) and T1w-SE sequences shows a high sensitivity in the detection of plasmacytoma manifestations with a relatively low specificity. Whole-body MRI is therefore suitable as an examination method in therapy monitoring in the case of identified plasmacytoma [17]. In current studies, the value of whole-body MRI compared to whole-body multisection CT is under investigation, especially with regard to costs and investment in time (Fig. 5.3).

5.3.1.4 Lymphoma

In approximately 20% of cases of Hodgkin lymphoma and up to 40% of non-Hodgkin lymphoma, a skeletal manifestation occurs, whereby this predominantly affects the spinal column, pelvis, ribs and proximal femur.

Both osteosclerotic and osteolytic lesions may present with very variable X-ray morphology. Analogous to metastases and plasmacytomas, MRI also shows high sensitivity here in the detection of lymphoma localization, although with low specificity, and is outstandingly suitable for the assessment of bone marrow complications (fracture risk). In a feasibility study conducted by Iizuka-Mikami et al. from 2004 [2], the options for detecting a bone marrow infiltration were compared in 34 patients with non-Hodgkin lymphoma between whole-body MRI, bone scintigraphy, and biopsy. The authors point out the high sensitivity of MRI in the detection of bone marrow infiltration, especially using STIR sequences, and primarily recommend the use of whole-body MRI for patients for whom it is not possible to perform a PET-CT. However, the use of whole-body MRI compared with other methods, such as multi-slice CT and PET-CT, in the diagnosis of bone dissemination still remains to be validated in further studies.

5.3.1.5 Further bone diseases

In the multifocal bone diseases described as follows, the use of whole-body MRI is suited for primary staging and for follow-up examinations in already identified disease, as well as in the search for a suitable biopsy region to verify the diagnosis:
- eosinophilic granuloma,
- chronic recurrent multifocal osteomylitis,
- Paget's disease,

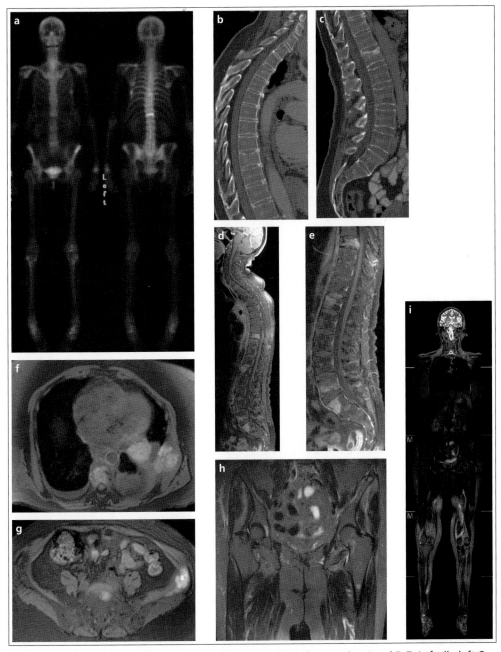

Figure 5.2a–i Melanoma metastases. Metastases T-spine 8 and 12, L-spine 4 and 5, 7. Left rib, left Os ilium, left Femur. **(a)** Bone scintigraphy; **(b, c)** 16-slice CT – sagittal reconstructions of the T/L-spine; **(d–i)** Whole-body MRI: sagittal T1w-SE-fatsat of T/L-spine and axial T1w-SE-fatsat thorax/abdomen following i.v. contrast agent, coronal TIRM of the pelvis, coronal TIRM whole-body overview.

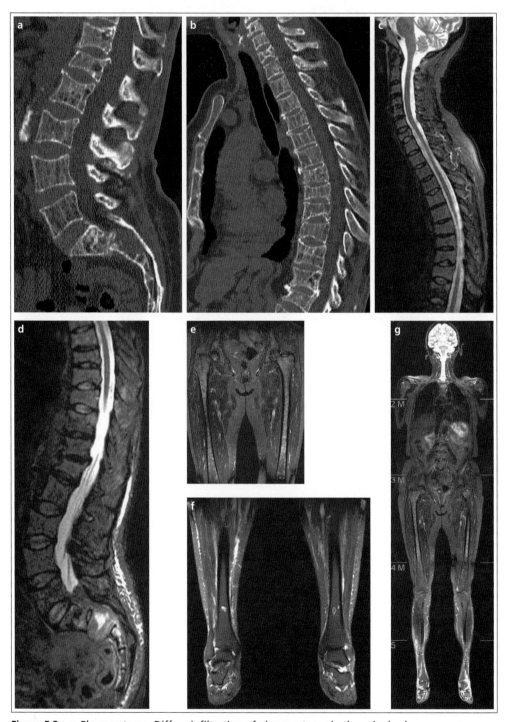

Figure 5.3a–g Plasmacytoma. Diffuse infiltration of plasmacytoma in the spinal column, sacrum, upper and lower legs, shoulders. **(a, b)** 16-slice spiral CT of the L/T-spine with sagittal reconstructions; **(c–g)** Whole-body MRI, sagittal and coronal TIRM.

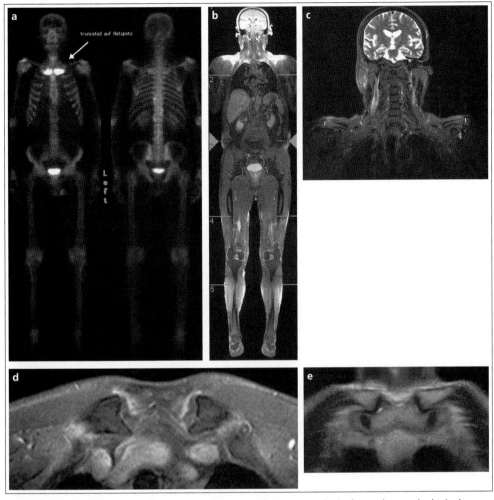

Figure 5.4a–e SAPHO syndrome. Typical infiltration of the sternoclavicular and acromioclavicular joints bilaterally. **(a)** Whole-body scintigraphy; **(b–e)** Whole-body MRI: coronal TIRM, T1w-SE, T1w-SE-fatsat post i.v. CA.

- SAPHO syndrome (pustulous arthroosteitis) (Fig. 5.4),
- musculoskeletal development disorders: especially osteochondrodysplasias, polyostotic fibrous dysplasia, multiple cartilaginous exostosis.

There are no extensive whole-body MRI studies on these disease groups in the current literature. Initial results, however, show the suitability of the method, especially for progress monitoring in young patients while providing the option of detecting disease complications and transformation tendencies.

5.3.2 Joints

Due to its ability to effectively depict the internal joint structures and periarticular soft tissue, MRI has progressed to become the method of choice in the diagnosis of individual joints. With the introduction of new techniques in whole-body MRI, new possibilities also arise in the diagnosis of polyarthritic diseases. Using the whole-body coil system, whole-body MRI offers resolution of the large joints with good detail. The small joints of the hand and foot, as well as the elbow joint, can only be generally evaluated, so that if high resolution imaging is required, e.g. for rheumatoid arthritis, an additional separate examination with a dedicated surface coil is necessary. A further problem arises in adipose patients in the imaging of the shoulder joint on the margins of the maximum field of view.

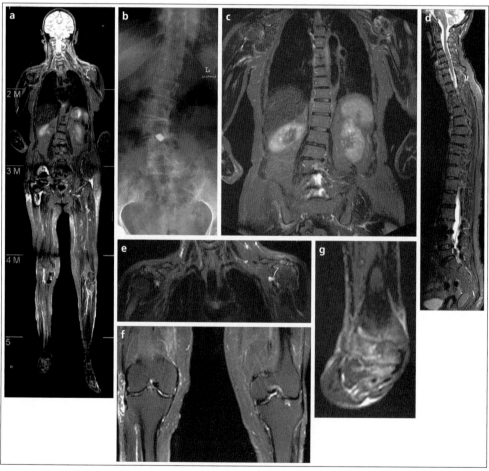

Figure 5.5a–g Rheumatoid arthritis. Acute infiltration of the lower cervical spine and the AC joint left; ankle joint right. Secondary result: Total hip replacement right; spondylosis L4/5. **(a)** Whole-body MRI: TIRM overview; **(b)** X-ray of lumbar spine ap; **(c–g)** Whole-body MRI: coronal and sagittal TIRM, coronal T1w-SE-fatsat following i.v. contrast agent.

With the aid of whole-body MRI, early arthritic changes in the large joints and spinal column can be efficiently imaged. Especially in young patients, whole-body MRI can replace repeated X-ray checks, with the exception of the hand and foot regions.

5.3.2.1 Rheumatoid arthritis

Rheumatoid arthritis is a systemic inflammatory connective tissue disease of unclear origin with chronic synovialitic joint destruction. The incidence is around 1% of the population. The disease starts in the metacarpophalangeal and interphalangeal joints of the fingers and

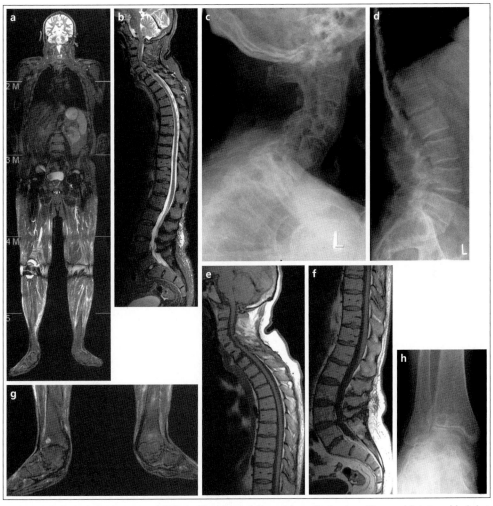

Figure 5.6a–h Ankylosing spondylitis. Infiltration of the mid cervical spine, iliosacral joint, ankle joint – non-acute; Secondary result: slight local metal artifacts due to total hip replacement bilaterally. **(a)** Whole-body MRI: coronal TIRM overview; **(b)** Whole-body MRI: sagittal TIRM whole-spine overview; **(c, d)** X-ray of C/L-spine lat.; **(e, f)** Whole-body MRI: sagittal T1w-SE of the C/L-spine; **(g)** Whole-body MRI: coronal TIRM of both ankle joints; **(h)** X-ray right ankle joint ap.

toes. Primary diagnostics usually involve determination of the rheumatoid factors, the typical clinical symptoms (ARA criteria), and X-ray diagnostics.

The potential of whole-body MRI is mainly to be seen in propagation diagnostics and progress monitoring in case of centripetal infiltration and of occipitocervical transition. The use of T1w spin-echo sequences with fat suppression following intravenous administration of contrast agent is important for presenting the pannus tissue (Fig. 5.5).

5.3.2.2 Ankylosing spondylitis (Bechterew disease)

Ankylosing spondylitis is one of the seronegative forms of spondylarthritis and shows a typical "mixed picture" of joint destruction, subchondral sclerosis and ankylosis, mainly in the region of the thoracolumbal transition of the spinal column and the iliosacral joints.

Peripherally, there is increased symmetrical infiltration of the hip joints, knee joints and shoulder joints, as well as of the manubriosternal joint.

Whole-body MRI can also be utilized as part of staging examinations to search for early changes, as well as in follow-up examinations. An advantage exists in the region of the spinal column, particularly in the detection of complications (Fig. 5.6).

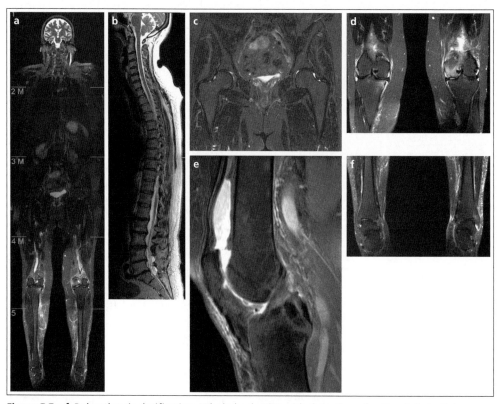

Figure 5.7a–f Polyarthrosis clarification. Whole-body MRI with detection of arthrosis in both knee joints and of the left AC joint; osteochondrosis of the L-spine. **(a)** Coronal TIRM whole-body overview; **(b)** sagittal TIRM whole-spine overview; **(c–f)** specific coronal and sagittal TIRM of hip, knee joint and ankle joints.

5.3.2.3 *Polyarthrosis and other diseases of the joints*

Whole-body MRI is also suitable for diagnostics of the large joints in the case of polyarthrosis (Fig. 5.7) and for joint conditions concurrent with systemic inflammatory connective tissue diseases, such as lupus erythematosus and scleroderma.

5.3.3   Muscular system

5.3.3.1 *Polymyositis/dermatomyositis*

Polymyositis is an inflammatory disease of the muscle with a symmetrical pattern of occurrence, in which additional dissemination in the skin (dermatomyositis) and joints (20 to 50% of cases) may occur. In 7% of polymyositides, there is an underlying connective tissue disease or a malignant disease. Differential diagnostic discrimination from a viral myositis, myasthenia gravis and motor neuron disease is important in the initial diagnosis. Given unspecific electromyographic results, frequent false-negative muscle enzymes in serum, and false-negative muscle biopsies in 10–25% of cases [6], a high potential arises for whole-body muscle diagnostics by means of MRI.

The use of coronal and axial TIRM sequences is generally sufficient to assess disease extent during initial diagnostics or acute exacerbation. T1-weighted spin-echo sequences can be called upon to differentiate between myositis and steroid-induced myopathy in patients who have already undergone treatment and to assess dystrophic muscle changes. In initial diagnostics, additional T1-weighted, fat suppressed sequences following admission of intravenous contrast agent are recommended to exclude primary tumors if tumor imaging diagnostics have not yet been performed. Whole-body MRI is outstandingly well suited for polymyositis diagnostics in general (Fig. 5.8).

5.3.3.2 *Muscular dystrophy/muscular hypertrophy*

Duchenne muscular dystrophy is an X-chromosome recessive inherited disease leading to the destruction of muscular tissue with subsequent replacement by fat and fibrous tissue. The first signs of the disease appear starting at an age of 3 years. There is a loss of muscle mass of approx. 4% per year during the course of the disease. Accurate quantification of the muscle loss and fatty tissue increase is important for the clinician. Work conducted by Pichiecchio et al. from the year 2000 [12] introduced a model to quantify the fat/muscle mass of the body in 9 children with Duchenne dystrophy using MRI with axial T1w spin-echo sequences on a 0.5 Tesla system. The authors recommend their very time-consuming method for monitoring the progress of the disease and for dietary planning. In a study from 2000 [14], Gong et al. recommend the inclusion of the Cavalieri method for volumetric assessment of the muscle and fat compartments in MRI. Using axial T1w spin-echo sequences, this study compared the volume distribution of the respective body compartments of 4 Duchenne patients with control groups.

A more experimental application of muscle-fat determination using whole-body MRI arises for the field of sports medicine (see Chap. 10). In a volunteer study from 2003, Abe et al. succeeded in ascertaining that after a 16-week weight training program, the skeletal muscle mass had increased more than the other fat-free body mass, whereby the muscular

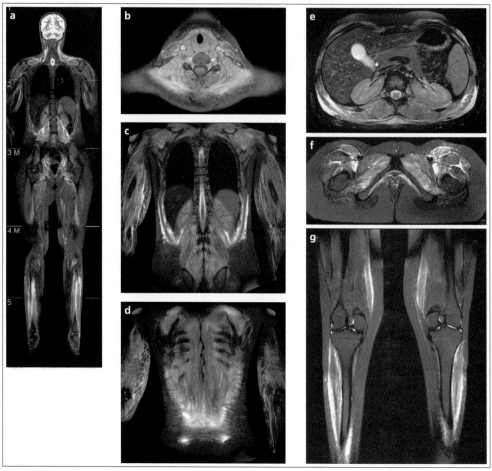

Figure 5.8a–g Polymyositis. Acute exacerbation of polymyositis with extended symmetric infiltration in the muscles of the trunk and the extremities. **(a–g)** Whole-body MRI with whole-body TIRM overview as well as specific coronal and axial TIRM sequences over the respective regions of the body.

hypertrophy was incident in varying degrees. This provides interesting perspectives for the investigation of the muscle structure and training success in athletes using whole-body MRI.

The basic requisite for muscle quantification is the acquisition of axial T1w sequences of the whole body. The measurement time for data acquisition is significantly reduced with the introduction of whole-body MRI technology, and the examination complexity is simultaneously reduced. Which evaluation method is to be preferred remains to be clarified in comparative studies. The muscle-fat volume determination of the body using whole-body MRI is generally reserved for special indications.

Bibliography

1. Engelhard K, Hollenbach HP, Wolfart K, von Imhoff E, Fellner FA. Comparison of whole-body MRI with automatic moving table technique and bone scintipraphy for screening for bone metastases in patients with breast cancer. Eur Radiol 2004; 14 (1): 99–105.

2. Iizuka-Mikami M, Nagai K, Yoshida K, Sugihara T, Suetsugu Y, Mikami M, Tamada T, Imai S, Kajihara Y, Fukunaga M. Detection of bone marrow and extramedullary involvement on patients with non-Hodgkin's lymphoma by whole-body MRI: comparison with bone and (67)Ga scintigraphics. Eur Radiol 2004; 14(6): 1074–81.

3. Mazumdar A, Siegel MJ, Narra V, Luchtman-Jones L. Whole body fast inversion recovery MR imaging of small cell neoplasms in pediatric patients: a pilot study. Am J Roentgenol 2002; 179(5): 1261–6.

4. Green RA, Saifuddin A. Whole spine MRI in the assessment of acute vertebral body trauma. Skeletal Radiol 2004; 33(3): 129–35.

5. Daldrup-Link HE, Franzius C, Link TM, Laukamp D, Sciuk J, Jurgens H, Schober O, Rummeny EJ. Whole body MR imaging for detection of bone metastases in children and young adults: comparison with bone scintigraphy and FDG PET. Am J Roentgenol 2001; 177(1): 229–36.

6. O'Connell MJ, Powell T, Brennan D, Lynch T, Mc Carthy CJ, Eustace SJ. Whole body MR imaging in the diagnosis of polymyositis. Am J Roentgenol 2002; 179(4): 967–71.

7. Walker RE, Eustace SJ. Whole body magnetic resonance imaging: techniques, clinical indications, and future applications. Semin Musculoskelet Radiol 2001; 5(1): 5–20.

8. Abe T, Kojima K, Kearns CF, Yohena H, Fukuda J. Whole body muscle hypertrophy from resistance training: distribution and total mass. Br J Sports Med 2003; 37(6): 543–5.

9. Gruning T, Tiepolt C, Kropp J, Franke WG. Diagnosis of bone metastasis with whole body MRI? Radiologe 2001; 41(9): 792–5.

10. Tausig A, Mantey N, Berger F, Sommer H, Pluger T, Hahn K. Advantages and limitations of whole-body bone marrow MRI using Turbo-STIR sequences in comparison to planar bone scans. Nuklearmedizin 2000; 39(6): 174–9.

11. Hargarden G, O'Connell M, Kavanagh E, Powell T, Ward R, Eustace S. Current concepts in whole-body imaging using turbo short tau inversion recovery MR imaging. Am J Roentgenol 2003; 180(1): 247–52.

12. Pichiecchio A, Uggetti C, Egitto MG, Berardinelli A, Orcesi S, Gorni KO, Zanardi C, Tagliabue A. Quantitative MR evaluation of body compistion in patients with Duchenne muscular dystrophy. Eur Radiol 2002; 12(11): 2704–9.

13. Lauenstein TC, Goedhe SC, Herborn CU, Treder W, Ruehm SG, Debatin JF, Barkhausen J. Three dimensional volumetric interpolated breath-hold MR imaging for whole-body tumor staging in less than 15 minutes: a feasibility study. Am J Roentgenol 2002; 179(2): 445–9.

14. Gong QY, Pheonix J, Kemp GJ, Garcia-Finana M, Frostick SP, Brodie DA, Edwards RH, Whitehouse GH, Roberts N. Estimation of body composition in muscular dystrophy by MRI and stereology. J Magn Reson Imaging 2000; 12(3): 467–75.

15. Bohndorf K, Imhof H. Radiologische Diagnostik der Knochen und Gelenke. Georg Thieme Verlag, Stuttgart, 1998.

16. Steinborn M, Tilling R, Heuck A, Brügel M, Stäbler A, Reiser M. Diagnostik der Metastasierung im Knochenmark mittels MRT. Radiologe 2000; 40: 826–834.

17. Baur A, Stabler A, Nagel D, Lamerz R, Bartl R, Hiller E, Wendtner C, Bachner F, Reiser M. Magnetic resonance imaging as a supplement for the clinical staging system of Durie and Salmon? Cancer 2002; 95(6): 1334–45.

18. Goehde S, Forsting M, Debatin J. Screening with MRI. A new "all inclusive" protocol. Semin Ultrasound CT MR 2003; 24: 2–11.

6 Whole-body MRI compared with bone scintigraphy and ^{18}F-FDG-PET in the detection of bone metastases

Nadir Ghanem

6.1 Introduction

After the lungs and the liver, the skeletal system is the third most common region of localization of distant metastases with malignant tumors. Depending on the various primary tumors, solid tumors show a relatively high rate of metastasis in the skeletal system [1]. The initial localization of metastasis in the skeletal system of patients with solid tumors takes place in the bone marrow. The prognosis for metastasis in the bone marrow is more favorable than for visceral metastasis. Screening of bone marrow metastases allows fast, targeted therapy with a concomitant reduction in morbidity. Autoptic studies indicate that the actual incidence of bone metastases with various solid malignant primary tumors is higher than the detection rate with radiological or nuclear medicine based techniques [2].

Nuclear medicine methods are of great importance in the diagnosis of bone metastases. The use of bone scintigraphy with technetium-marked phosphate complexes has been largely unrivalled in the basic diagnostics of bone metastases since the 1980s, and this method of examination, with its sensitivity in excess of 95%, has been shown to be an effective screening examination for malignant solid tumors [3, 4].

However, the significance of bone scintigraphy has become overshadowed in recent years, as major studies have demonstrated that bone metastases can be detected even at early stages of infiltration using MRI, before scintigraphic detection succeeds [5–8].

Positron emission tomography (PET) is increasingly used successfully in whole-body staging, which also covers the skeletal system, as an imaging modality for bone metastasis. Combined PET/CT has come of age over the last couple of years in the diagnosis and staging of oncological patients [12, 13].

MRI is now superior in its sensitivity, specificity and in diagnosing the extent of bone metastasis, to scintigraphy, which is now over 30 years old. As a very sensitive technique, it reveals bone metastasis in the axial skeleton and the peripheral skeletal system [14–20]. Possible threatening complications of bone metastasis in the spinal column can be easily detected with MRI [5, 20]. Its greatest limitation was a limited examination field of view, such that whole-body depiction required multiple examinations using different coils and consequently relatively long examination times [8].

New developments in MRI, such as ultrafast data acquisition and new coil and moving table concepts, today allow the performance of a whole-body examination within a tolerable and considerably reduced examination time [22–25].

For bone metastasis diagnostics with whole-body MRI, there are only a few studies available with small case numbers and a partly inhomogeneous patient population [8, 22–27].

The aim of this article is to present the importance of MRI and whole-body MRI in comparison with the established techniques of bone scintigraphy and ^{18}F-FDG-PET in the detection of bone metastases.

6.2 The occurrence and distribution patterns of bone metastases

Bone metastases are 25 times more common than primary bone tumors: Three different metastasis progressions are possible in principle. Besides per-continuitatem infiltration and lymphatic protraction, the bloodstream represents by far the most significant means of propagation in the form of hematogenic dissemination.

The relative frequency of bone metastases varies dependent on the respective metastasis type; for example, with the pulmonary type, metastases occur in 34% of cases, followed by the cava type with 25% and the portal type with 7% [28].

Bone metastases predominantly occur in hematopoietically active bone marrow, which in adults is primarily located in the bones of the trunk as well as the skull and the proximal regions of the humeri and femura [29]. This ultimately leads to the preferred metastasis localization in the axial skeleton (80%), the femura (40%), and the skull and pelvis (20%). Other sites of manifestation are the ribs and the sternum (25–30%) [29].

6.3 Bone scintigraphy and ^{18}F-FDG-PET in the detection of bone metastases

Nuclear medicine methods are of great importance in the diagnosis of bone metastases. The use of bone scintigraphy with technetium-marked phosphate complexes has been largely unrivalled since the 1980s in the basic diagnostics of bone metastases, and, with its sensitivity in excess of 95%, it has also been shown to be an effective screening examination for malignant solid tumors [3, 4, 29]. The use of 'regions of interest', of SPECT (single photon emission computed tomography) technology, and of multiphase bone scintigraphy have led to an increase in the already high sensitivity of the examination technique and in particular to an increase in the specificity of bone scintigraphy.

However, the significance of bone scintigraphy has become overshadowed in recent years, as major studies have demonstrated that bone metastases can be detected even at early stages of dissemination using MRI, before scintigraphic detection succeeds [5–8].

Bone scintigraphy currently remains the most conclusive and cost-effective technique to allow a whole-body examination of almost all patients with high sensitivity [19–21, 29].

Compared with conventional X-ray overview examinations, bone scintigraphy is certainly a more sensitive technique. Furthermore, the time interval between the positive bone scintillation result and the subsequent positive X-ray result shows a difference of several months [30]. The effective dosage of bone scintigraphy using ^{99m}Tc-marked polyphosphonates with an application of 555 to 740 MBq of activity is around 4 mSv. Numerous studies confirm the sensitivity of bone scintigraphy in the detection of bone metastases [29–32]. On the other hand, a frequently cited limitation is the low specificity [29, 30]. The phosphonates are not only enriched in malignant processes, but especially also in the inflammation accompanying arthritides and osteomyelitides, in trauma, and in benign bone tumors. Given knowledge of the full clinical information and drawing upon conventional X-ray diagnostics, the specificity of bone scintigraphy can be raised to 95% [33]. Three-dimensional imaging of the skeletal system in SPECT technology raises the specificity of bone scintigraphy, as this technique presents significantly improved anatomical localization of the enrichment detected by scintigraphy.

For this reason, PET has now become established as a more modern nuclear medicine technique for clinical routine work, and, alongside ^{18}F-FDG-PET, ^{18}F-fluoride-PET has also arrived in the detection of bone metastases [9, 10, 19, 29, 34, 35]. ^{18}F-FDG-PET (fluorodeoxyglucose) is used most frequently in oncological diagnostics. This PET tracer is a marker for cellular glucose metabolism and is significantly enhanced in malignomas. ^{18}F-FDG is not tumor specific, rather it is partly also enriched in inflamed tissue. Initial studies in which the value of bone scintigraphy is compared with that of ^{18}FDG-PET present divergent results. However, bone metastases can be significantly more effectively excluded using PET, as degenerative changes in the bone are not presented to the same extent in ^{18}FDG-PET as in bone scintigraphy [10, 11, 34, 35].

PET offers advantages over bone scintigraphy in that the technique is, on the one hand, a purely tomographic acquisition technique and, on the other hand, the local resolution of PET is much higher than that of bone scintigraphy. Besides ^{18}F-FDG, ^{18}F-fluoride is increasingly used as an osteotropic radiotracer, which shows a greater bone uptake than ^{99m}Tc-marked biophosphonates and also, by virtue of increased renal clearance, leads to an improved contrast between compact and trabecular bone [34]. Comparing ^{18}FDG-PET with bone scintigraphy, it is apparent that ^{18}FDG-PET shows greater sensitivity than planar scintigraphy [35–38]. In contrast, some studies show that ^{18}FDG-PET is less sensitive than bone scintigraphy in the detection of bone metastases in prostate carcinoma and osteogenic sarcoma [10, 39].

Comparing the number of detected lesions in 145 patients with different primary tumors, the sensitivity is higher with ^{18}FDG-PET than with bone scintigraphy [40]. These results are confirmed in patients with breast carcinoma. In a differential analysis, the superiority of bone scintigraphy was shown in the sub-group of female patients with purely osteoblastic metastases [11]. Schirrmeister et al. compared ^{18}F-fluoride-PET with bone scintigraphy, and ^{18}F-fluoride-PET detected a total of 64 bone metastases in 17 out of 34 patients [34]. With bone scintigraphy only 11 out of 34 patients were positive, with a total of 29 metastases.

6.4 Bone (marrow) metastases in MRI

Metastasis propagation in the bone marrow leads to an increase in T1 relaxation times with consequent signal decay compared with T1-weighted imaging in the high signal fatty tissue. Changes in the T2-weighted relaxation time differ. There is an increase in the T2 time with a significant signal increase of the lesion; solid, cell-rich tumor regions show an intermediate signal intensity in T2-weighted imaging. However, given accompanying osteoblastic components and bone regeneration, the T2 relaxation time drops again and there is a fall in signal intensity of the lesion in T2-weighted imaging. In principle, it should be said that malignant, as well as inflammatory bone marrow, conditions lead to signal attenuation due to an increase in the amount of water and suppression of the fat components in T1-weighted imaging. T1-weighted spin-echo sequences are therefore an essential aspect in the detection of bone marrow metastases. They should be supplemented with T2-weighted sequences with fat suppression, such as the STIR technique or with sequence-selective, fat suppressed T2-weighted sequences [41]. As a consequence of fat suppression of normal bone marrow and the emphasis on T2 prolongation due to pathological infiltration, these sequences achieve an especially high contrast between the lesion and the normal healthy fatty marrow [42].

Phase-shifted gradient-echo imaging – unenhanced and contrast-enhanced – was found to be very sensitive as a search sequence in metastasis detection [43, 44]. Administration of intravenous contrast agent is not of great assistance in the detection and characterization of bone metastases. The application of contrast agent can depict extraosseous (paraosseous/paravertebral/intraspinal) soft tissue tumor components in order to demonstrate the precise extent of the tumor and thereby reveal potentially threatening complications [5, 42–44].

In the case of malignant underlying diseases, enhanced reconversion of the bone marrow may occur due to the disease or in association with the therapy [45]. The hemopoietically active bone marrow is characterized in T1-weighted imaging by a low signal and in T2 or STIR imaging by a higher signal than the adjacent normal fatty marrow. Hematopoietically active bone marrow regions can be configured irregularly or arranged focally, so that they are very difficult to distinguish from the skeletal/bone metastases in their differential diagnosis. The use of opposed-phase gradient-echo sequences was shown to be very helpful in the detection of hematopoietic marrow [46, 47].

6.5 The value of MRI compared with bone scintigraphy and ^{18}F-FDG-PET

The detection of bone metastasis in tumor patients is of enormous clinical significance for stage classification and the resulting therapy planning [5, 44]. Localization and propagation of bone metastasis must be depicted to identify potentially threatening complications of bone metastasis in a timely manner. Since the beginning of the 1990s, it is well known that MRI succeeds in detecting bone marrow involvement at an early stage, before bone scintigraphy can detect any bone involvement [5, 8, 9, 14, 15, 18, 48–50].

The sensitivity of MRI in the detection of metastases is cited as up to 100% in the literature [51]. In numerous studies, MRI was consistently evaluated as superior to bone scintigraphy [5, 7, 8, 14, 48–55]. Many studies have reported a higher sensitivity for MRI based on a patient comparison [5, 18, 53, 54] as well as a regional comparison [5, 15, 16, 44].

At the beginning of the 1990s, Frank et al. reported on 95 patients with bone metastasis; 30 of the 95 patients (28%) showed no metastases with bone scintigraphy, whereas MRI detected bone metastases in all the patients [14]. Avrahami et al. underlined the enormous advantage of MRI compared with bone scintigraphy in a study of 10 patients with small-cell bronchial carcinoma [53].

Haubold-Reuter et al. studied 21 patients with malignant underlying diseases and showed clear superiority of MRI compared with bone scintigraphy in the axial skeleton [15]. Only 70% of the lesions seen with MRI were detected in bone scintigraphy. The authors nevertheless pointed out the fact that in 11 of 21 patients bone scintigraphy detected lesions outside the MRI examination field of view, which certainly represents a major limitation of MRI [5, 7, 8, 15, 44].

In a comparative study conducted by Altehoefer et al., peripheral bone metastases were described in 26 out of 81 patients with bone scintigraphy, but MRI of the axial skeleton was markedly superior to bone scintigraphy [5]. Altehoefer et al. examined a total of 81 breast carcinoma patients and showed a clear superiority of MRI over bone scintigraphy in regard to detection and propagation of metastases in the axial skeleton [5]. The result for bone scintigraphy was false-negative for seven of the 81 patients. For 26 out of 53 patients with positive concordant results (49%), MRI showed more extensive disease with a subsequent therapeutic consequence. The greatest limitation of this comparative study is the fact that only a few positive lesions found in the study were verified histologically.

Besides its superiority in the detection and propagation diagnostics of bone metastasis, MRI, as an imaging technique, is in a position to present additional results from the axial skeleton which are of relevance for therapy [5, 17, 29, 44, 55]. Altehoefer et al. reported over 81 secondary results visible in MRI among 45 female breast carcinoma patients with positive concordant results in MRI and bone scintigraphy in the axial skeleton: Vertebral posterior border involvement (n = 22), vertebral arch (n = 16), pathological vertebral fractures (n = 18), spinal canal constriction (n = 14), myelon compression (n = 11). For 28 out of 45 breast carcinoma female patients, the MRI result led to a change in the therapy regime [5]. Direct comparisons between MRI and ¹⁸FDG-PET are available only in a few studies. In a study directly comparing three different modalities (whole-body MRI, ¹⁸FDG-PET, and bone scintigraphy) in a total of 39 children and youths, Daldrup-Link et al. reported clear superiority of ¹⁸FDG-PET with a sensitivity of 90% compared with MRI. Bone scintigraphy was well behind with a sensitivity of 71% [35].

In a retrospective study of 38 patients, Ghanem et al. demonstrated eight discordant results between MRI and PET in the axial skeleton. In seven out of eight cases, ¹⁸FDG-PET was false-negative, and in two out of 7 cases a change in therapy regime followed. In one case the MRI was false-negative [56].

6.6 Whole-body MRI in the detection of bone metastases

Previous limitations of MRI in clinical routine work were due to a restricted examination field of view, so that several examinations using different coils were required to present the whole body [7, 8, 43, 57, 68]. The development of ultra-fast data acquisition for MRI high performance gradient systems with fast slew rates has recently allowed whole-body MRI to be performed within a tolerable time [8, 12, 22–27, 35, 57–65, 68, 69, 71–74].

With the development of the moving table technique using a whole-body table top (An-gioSURF [System for Unlimited Rolling Field of Views, MR-Innovation, Essen, Germany]) it has become possible to perform whole-body MR-examinations for clinical routine use [12, 24, 60, 62, 63] (Fig. 6.1–6.4) (also see Chap. 7). In our own whole-body examinations with the AngioSURF system, 129 comparisons with bone scintigraphy were possible [24]. In 56 out of 129 patients (43%), typical metastasis lesions were not found, either with whole-body MRI or with scintigraphy. In 49 out of 129 patients (38%), both examination techniques were positive in detecting bone metastases (Fig. 6.2, 6.4, 6.5). Investigating the extent of the bone metastasis in 49 patients with positive concordant results in the axial skeleton, as well as in the peripheral skeletal system, it was possible to detect a similar extent of skeletal metastasis in 21 out of 49 patients (43%). In 22 out of 49 patients with positive concordant results (45%), whole-body MRI was superior to bone scintigraphy (Fig. 6.2, 6.4); in 6 out of 49 cases, bone scintigraphy was superior to whole-body imaging (12%).

In 24 patients (19%) there were discordant results in the detection of bone metastases (Fig. 6.1). In 15 out of 129 patients (12%), whole-body MRI examinations revealed bone metastases, whereas bone scintigraphy failed to detect any changes typical of metastases in either the axial skeleton or in the peripheral skeletal system. In one case, however, whole-body MRI was false-positive in the detection of a unifocal signal intensity increase in the thoracic spine, which, when viewed together with a CT, represented a hemangioma, but

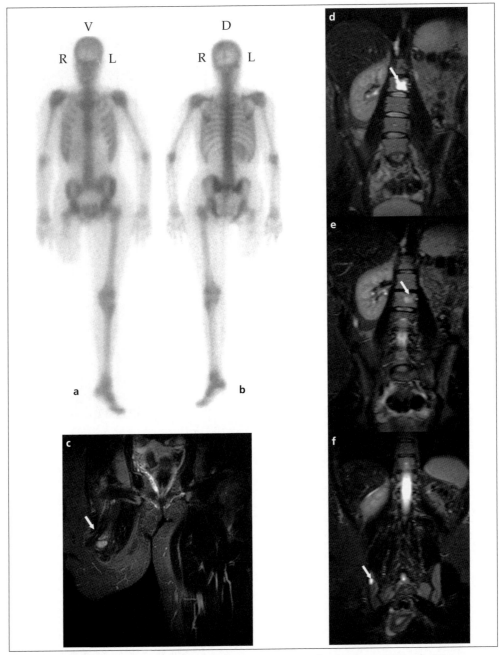

Figure 6.1a–f 34-year-old female patient in the follow-up examination for a PNET (primitive neuro-ectodermal tumor).

(a, b) The bone scintigraphy (with kind permission: Prof. Dr. Dr. Dr. h.c. E. Moser, Dept. of Nuclear Medicine, University Hospital Freiburg, Germany) shows neither increased uptake of the radiophar-maceutical in the anterior and posterior projections nor a photopenic defect.

(c–f) The whole-body MRI performed at the same time detects four skip lesions in the L-spine, the pelvis and the remaining right upper leg stump in the form of metastases (arrow).

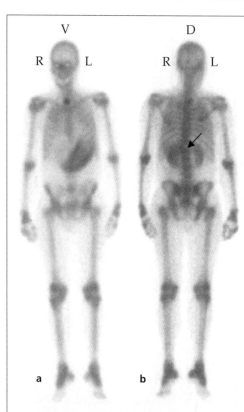

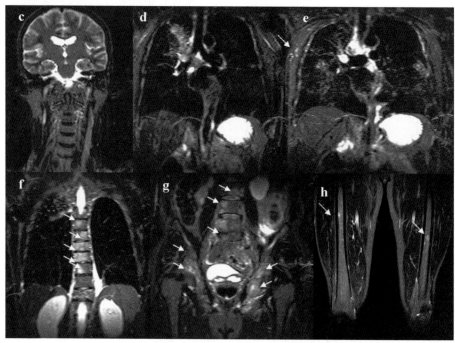

Figure 6.2a–h 64-year-old patient with bronchial carcinoma.

(a, b) The bone scintigraphy (with kind permission: Prof. Dr. Dr. Dr. h. c. E. Moser, Dept. of Nuclear Medicine, University Hospital Freiburg, Germany) in the posterior projection shows a photopenic defect in the lower T-spine (arrow) indicative of a bone metastasis.

(c–h) Whole-body MRI shows a diffuse, partly multifocal metastasis in the axial skeleton and in the peripheral skeletal system (arrow) and is therefore clearly superior to bone scintigraphy. The primary tumor with lymphogenous metastasis is also depicted **(d, e)**.

the whole-body MRI was able to correctly detect a progressive femur metastasis. The bone scintigraphy performed at the same time was negative. In 14 out of 15 cases whole-body MRI was shown to be true positive in the detection of bone metastases in the axial and peripheral skeletal system, with the exception of the hemangioma diagnosed as a metastatic site.

In nine cases (7%), bone scintigraphy was superior to whole-body MRI; in all cases unifocal metastases in the axial skeleton or in the peripheral skeletal system were present. In two of the nine cases the diagnosis was not verified in the course of the study. In three cases, progress in the condition could be conclusively shown over the course of the study with nuclear medicine and radiological examination techniques, so that there were false-negative MRI results in three out of nine cases. Since the end of 2003, a new whole-body coil system equipped with 76 coil elements and 32 radiofrequency channels has been offered in a 1.5 Tesla system (Magnetom Avanto, Siemens Medical Solutions, Erlangen, Germany) [58, 59, 64, 66, 67] (Fig. 6.5). In this new MRI system, coronal STIR imaging with a 205 cm field of view is possible within 14 minutes with good spatial resolution.

Eustace et al. were the first to compare whole-body MRI using turbo-STIR imaging with planar bone scintigraphy in 1997 [25].

A total of 25 patients with various tumor entities were studied; the authors determined a sensitivity for whole-body MRI of 96.5% and a specificity of 100%. Planar bone scintigraphy, as an established technique, has a sensitivity of 72% and a specificity of 98% [25].

Steinborn et al. studied 18 patients with different malignant underlying diseases and the suspicion of bone metastases with a study protocol comprising STIR imaging and T1-weighted spin-echo imaging [9]. The whole-body MRI detected 91.4% of the metastases verified and confirmed in the course of the study, whereas bone scintigraphy only detected 89 of the 105 lesions (85%).

Regarding the distribution pattern of anatomical localization in this study from Steinborn et al., whole-body MRI was a superior technique in the axial skeleton and in the extremities, whereas bone scintigraphy detected more lesions in the skull and thoracic skeleton, as expected [9]. This is partly reflected in our own study results [24, 69], in which whole-body MRI is regionally inferior to bone scintigraphy in the ribs.

In a study of 26 patients, Lauenstein et al. reported on a total of 60 regions that were detected with bone scintigraphy as metastasis infiltrated. Whole-body MRI was identical in 53 regions [26] (also see Chap. 7). The results not detected with whole-body MRI were in the region of the skull and ribs. This partially agrees with our own results [24, 67, 69] and those of other authors [35, 60, 62, 63, 67]. Goo et al. were, however, unable to confirm this in a study of 41 children.

Tausig et al. studied 20 female patients with breast carcinoma using a turbo-STIR sequence to exclude or detect bone metastases [65]. In 11 of the 20 patients (55%), both bone scintigraphy and whole-body MRI were positive, although bone scintigraphy only revealed 109 lesions in the skeletal system typical of metastasis, but whole-body MRI 150. The authors refer to the enormous limitations due to artifacts, in particular pulsation artifacts in the thorax, which hamper assessment of the ribs, sternum, and scapula. These were not confirmed by Goo et al. in a whole-body MRI study of children [71].

Lauenstein et al. underlined that the coronal orientation selected to depict long bones, such as the femur and humerus and the spinal column, can lead to disappointing detection results in the thoracic skeleton [26]. It was therefore proposed to image these skeletal regions with an axial orientation [63]. Engelhard et al. studied 22 female patients with breast carcinoma (coronal STIR sequences combined with axial T2-weighted TSE imaging of the head and T1-weighted opposed-phase imaging for the complete spinal column) [60]. In 12 of the 22 cases, both examination techniques were positive. In their study, the sensitivity for whole-body MRI was specified as 92%, whereas for bone scintigraphy sensitivity was shown to be 63%. The specificity for whole-body MRI was 90%, for bone scintigraphy 80%. The diagnostic accuracy was specified as 91% for whole-body MRI and 82% for bone scintigraphy [60]. For whole-body MRI, Goo et al. specified a sensitivity of 99% in the detection of bone metastases and a positive predictive value (PPV) of 94%, whereas bone scintigraphy achieved values of 26% and 76%, respectively. The authors compared whole-body MRI with 123-J-MIBG scintigraphy and showed a significant superiority of whole-body MRI in skeletal metastasis detection. Mentzel et al. detected 119 bone metastases with whole-body MRI using a STIR sequence; however, bone scintigraphy only detected 58 lesions (47%) [73].

There are still only limited data available to directly compare whole-body MRI, bone scintigraphy, and ^{18}FDG-PET [35, 67, 69, 72] (Fig. 6.3–6.5).

Daldrup-Link et al. studied 39 children and youths in direct comparison of whole-body MRI, ^{18}FDG-PET, and bone scintigraphy [35]. Clear superiority of ^{18}FDG-PET with a sensitivity of 90% was shown, whereas whole-body MRI using a T1-weighted and T2-weighted spin-echo sequence combined with STIR imaging showed a sensitivity of 82%. Bone scintigraphy produced a sensitivity of 71% [35]. In our own studies, whole-body MRI also

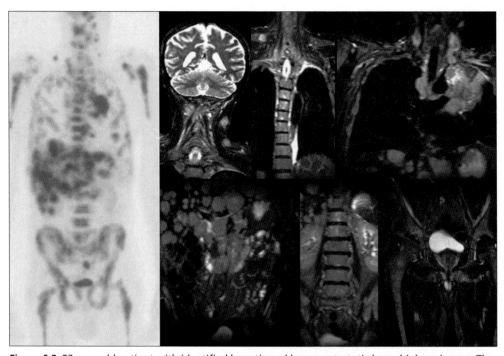

Figure 6.3 83-year-old patient with identified hepatic and bone metastatic bronchial carcinoma. The ^{18}F-FDG-PET (with kind permission: Prof. Dr. Dr. Dr. h. c. E. Moser, Dept. of Nuclear Medicine, University Hospital Freiburg, Germany) and whole-body MRI show, in addition to the diffuse bone metastasis in the axial skeleton, multifocal hepatic metastasis as well as cervical and medial lymphogenous metastasis with a left central tumor. ^{18}F-FDG-PET also presents a metastatic infiltration of the humeri.

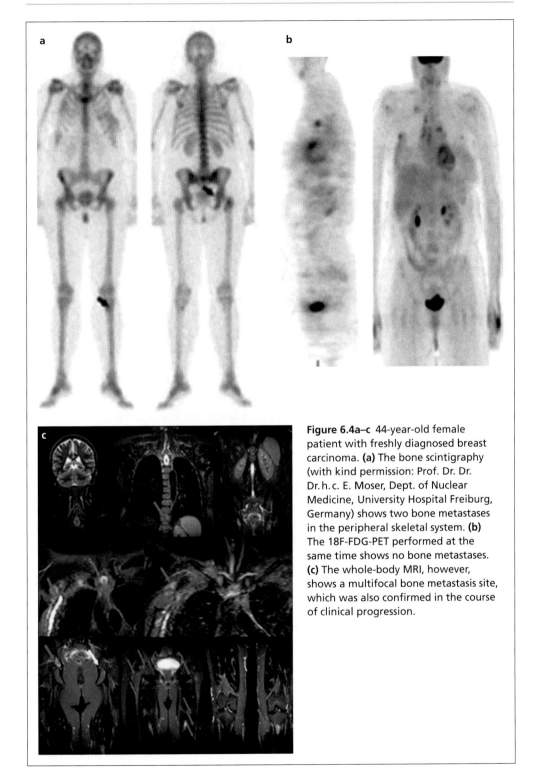

Figure 6.4a–c 44-year-old female patient with freshly diagnosed breast carcinoma. **(a)** The bone scintigraphy (with kind permission: Prof. Dr. Dr. Dr. h. c. E. Moser, Dept. of Nuclear Medicine, University Hospital Freiburg, Germany) shows two bone metastases in the peripheral skeletal system. **(b)** The 18F-FDG-PET performed at the same time shows no bone metastases. **(c)** The whole-body MRI, however, shows a multifocal bone metastasis site, which was also confirmed in the course of clinical progression.

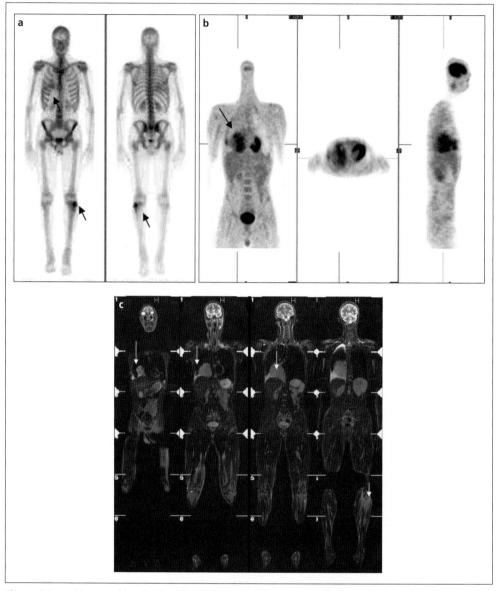

Figure 6.5a–c 26-year-old patient with a right central tumor, as well as paraosseous and osseous metastasis in the left lower leg. **(a)** Bone scintigraphy (with kind permission: Prof. Dr. Dr. Dr. h.c. E. Moser, Dept. of Nuclear Medicine, University Hospital Freiburg, Germany) shows a solitary metastasis in the left lower extremity and osseous involvement of the right ventral hemithorax (arrow). **(b)** ^{18}F-FDG-PET performed at the same time (with kind permission: Prof. Dr. Dr. Dr. h.c. E. Moser, Dept. of Nuclear Medicine, University Hospital Freiburg, Germany) shows the primary tumor as well as an adjacent pleural metastasis (arrow). **(c)** The whole-body MRI firstly shows the primary tumor with adjacent right-side pleural metastasis and effusion, and secondly the metastasis in the left dorsal tibia (arrow).

showed superiority over 1^{8}F-FDG-PET in the detection of bone metastases [67, 69, 72]. In 35 out of 130 cases (27%) there were positive concordant results (Fig. 6.3). In 85 patients, both techniques succeeded in excluding bone metastases, leading to total concordance in 92% of cases. In 3 cases ^{18}F-FDG-PET was superior to whole-body MRI, in 7 cases the reverse was the case [69] (Fig. 6.4, 6.5).

Numerous authors refer to secondary results associated with tumors which were detected with whole-body MRI as opposed to bone scintigraphy [24–27].

In our own study of 129 patients with solid tumors, whole-body MRI succeeded in presenting tumor-associated secondary results in 77 patients relating to the primary tumor, lymph node, soft tissue and distant metastasis in visceral organs [24] (Fig. 6.1, 6.5). In 52 of the 129 patients (40%), there were no tumor-relevant secondary results found with whole-body MRI. In 63 out of 129 patients, various primary tumors were detected, of which 52 cases were large bronchial carcinomas. In 54 out of 129 patients, lymph node enlargement was detected with a total number of 102 enlarged lymph node stations. In 30 of the 129 patients, distant metastasis in the liver (n = 21), lung (n = 6), adrenal glands (n = 4), and brain (n = 5) was shown. Secondary results associated with tumors in patients with negative concordant results between whole-body MRI and bone scintigraphy were recorded in 29 of the 48 (60%) patients with the help of whole-body MRI. Eighteen primary tumors were detected. In 17 patients, 39 lymph node enlargements were described. Soft tissue metastases associated with tumors were detected in 8 cases, and in 15 cases information on distant metastasis in the liver (n = 11), brain (n = 5), lung (n = 2), and adrenal glands (n = 1) was described.

Eustace et al. reported secondary findings in 13 out of 25 (52%) patients [25]. In their study of 17 breast carcinoma female patients, Walker et al. refer to liver lesions in 5 of 17 cases (29%) and CNS metastasis in 4 out of 17 cases (24%) [26]. In our own studies, secondary results associated with tumors of relevance to therapy were detected in 77 out of 129 cases (60%) by whole-body MRI.

Lauenstein et al. undertook a study of tumor-associated (n = 56) and non-tumor-associated secondary results (n = 36) [27]. The results associated with tumors largely comprised those from liver and lung metastases, which were detected with the STIR sequence in 47 out of 56 cases (84%). In the non-tumor-associated secondary results, T1-weighted gradient-echo imaging was most sensitive; the HASTE sequence was not shown to be very sensitive, either in relation to non-tumor-associated or tumor-associated conditions in patients with malignant underlying diseases and bone metastases.

Summarizing, it can be said that whole-body MRI represents a promising new staging technique for the detection of bone metastases in the oncological diagnosis of solid tumors, which in many cases is more sensitive than the established technique of bone scintigraphy in regard to the detection and extent of bone metastases in the entire skeletal system. The staging of rib metastases is problematic with whole-body MRI. Secondary results associated with tumors of relevance to therapy are detected with whole-body MRI.

There is still only a limited amount of partly contradictory data available comparing whole-body MRI with ^{18}FDG-PET in the detection of bone metastases, so that large comparative studies using special tracers and PET-CT are still outstanding. Whole-body MRI, as a new, fast, and effective examination method, offers significantly better detail presentation than bone scintigraphy and is easy to implement in clinical diagnostic routine work; due to the absence of radiation exposure, comprehensive progress monitoring is possible without reservations.

Bibliography

1. Nyström JS, Weiner JM, Heffeldinger-Juttner J. Metastatic and histologic presentation in unknown primary cancer. Semin Oncol 1977; 4: 53.
2. Abrams HL, Spiro R, Goldstein N. Metastases in carcinoma: analysis of 1000 autopsied cases. Cancer 1950; 3: 336–40.
3. Jacobson AF, Fogelman I. Bone Scanning in clinical oncology: does it have a future? Eur J Nucl Med 1998; 25: 1219–23.
4. Moser E. Die Bedeutung der Skelettszintigraphie in der Nachsorge von Malignompatienten. Radiologe 1990; 30: 465–71.
5. Altehoefer C, Ghanem N, Högerle S, Moser E, Langer M. Comparative detectability of bone metastases and impact on therapy of magnetic resonance imaging and bone scintigraphy in patients with breast cancer. Eur J Radiol 2001; 40: 16–23.
6. Layer G, Steudel A, Schüller H, van Kaick G, Grünwald F, Reiser M et al. MRI to detect bone marrow metastases in the initial staging of small cell lung carcinoma and breast carcinoma. Cancer 1999; 85: 1004–9.
7. Steinborn M, Tilling R, Heuck A, Brügel M, Stäbler A, Reiser M. Diagnostik der Metastasierung im Knochenmark mittels MRT. Radiologe 2000; 40: 826–34.
8. Steinborn MM, Heuck AF, Tiling R, Bruegel M, Gauger L, Reiser MF. Whole-body bone marrow MRI in patients with metastastic disease to skeletal system. J Comput Assit Tomogr 1999; 23: 123–9.
9. Brink I, Moser E. Nuklearmedizinische Diagnostik und Therapie: Sichere und effiziente Detektion von Skelettmetastasen. Klinikarzt 2000; 29: 276–80.
10. Franzius C, Sciuk J, Daldrup-Link HE, Jurgens H, Schober O. FDG-PET for detection of osseous metastases from malignant primary bone tumors: comparison with bone scintigraphy. Eur J Nucl Med 2000; 27: 1305–11.
11. Cook GJ, Houston S, Rubens R et al. Detection of bone metastases in breast cancer by 18 FDG-PET: different metabolic activity in osteoblastic and osteolytic lesions. J Clin Oncol 1998; 16: 3375–9.
12. Antoch G, Vogt FM, Freudenberg LS et al. Whole-body dual-modality PET/CT and whole-body MRI for tumor staging in oncology. JAMA 2003; 290: 3199–206.
13. Even-Sapir E, Metser U, Flusser G et al. Assessment of malignant skeletal disease: initial experience with 18F-Fluoride PET/CT and comparison between 18F-Fluoride PET and 18F-Fluoride PET/CT. J Nucl Med 2004; 45: 272–8.
14. Frank JA, Ling A, Patronas NJ, Carrasquillo JA, Horvath K, Hickey AM, Dwyer AJ. Detection of malignant bone tumors: MR imaging vs scintigraphy. AJR Am J Roentgenol 1990; 155: 1043–8.
15. Haubold-Reuter BG, Duewell S, Schilcher BR, Marincek B, von Schulthess GK. Musculoskeletal radiology: Fast spin echo MRI and bone scintigraphy in the detection of bone metastases. Eur Radiol 1993; 3: 316–20.
16. Sanal SM, Flickinger FW, Caudell MJ, Sherry RM. Detection of bone marrow involvement in breast cancer with magnetic resonance imaging. J Clin Oncol 1994; 12: 1415–21
17. Yamaguchi T. Intertrabecular vertebral metastases: metastases only detectable on MR imaging. Semin Musculoskelet Radiol 2001; 5: 171–5.
18. Jones AL, Williams MP, Powles TJ, Oliff JF, Hardy JR, Cherryman G, Husband J. Magnetic resonance imaging in the detection of bone metastases in patients with breast cancer. Br J Cancer 1990; 62: 296–8.
19. Cook GJ, Fogelman I. The role of nuclear medicine in monitoring treatment in skeletal malignancy. Semin Nucl Med 2001; 31: 206–11.
20. Mirza I, Cuello B, Ramachandran A, Johns W. Bone marrow biopsy and bone scan to detect skeletal malignancy. Semin Nucl Med 2001; 26: 677–9.
21. Rybak LD, Rosenthal DI Radiological imaging for the diagnosis of bone metastases. Q J Nucl Med 2001; 45: 53–64.

22. Eustace SJ, Walker R, Blake M, Yucel EK. Whole-body MR imaging: practical issues, clinical applications, and future directions. MRI Clinics of North America 1999; 7: 209–36.

23. Walker RE, Eustace SJ. Whole-body magnetic resonance imaging: techniques, clinical indications, and future applications. Semin Musculoskel Radiol 2001; 5: 5–20.

24. Ghanem N, Kelly T, Altehoefer C, et al. Whole-Body MRI in comparison to bone scintigraphy for detection of bone metastases in patients with solid tumors. Radiologe 2004; 44: 864–74.

25. Eustace S, Tello R, DeCarvalho V, Carey J, Melhem E, Yucel EK. A comparison of whole-body turboSTIR MR imaging and planar ^{99m}Tc-methylene diphosphonate scintigraphy in the examination of patients with suspected bone metastases. AJR Am J Roentgenol 1997; 169: 1655–61.

26. Lauenstein TC, Freudenberg LS, Goehde SC, Ruehm SG, Goyen M, Bosk S, Debatin JF, Barkhausen. J. Whole-body MRI using a rolling for detection of bone metastases. Eur Radiol 2002; 12: 2091–9.

27. Walker R, Kessar P, Blanchard K, Dimasi M, Harper K, DeCarvalho V, Yucel EK, Patriquin L, Eustace S. Turbo STIR magnetic resonance imaging as a whole-body screening tool for metastases in patients with breast carcinoma: Preliminary Clinical Experience. J Magn Reson Imaging 2000; 11: 343–50.

28. Adler CP, Herget G, Uhl M. Knochenmetastasen In: Adler CP, Herget G, Uhl M (Hrsg.) Radiologische Diagnostik der Knochenkrankheiten. Springer, Berlin, Heidelberg, New York, 2004, S. 166–70.

29. Hamaoka T, Madewell JE, Podoloff DA, Hortobagyi GN, Ueno NT. Bone imaging in metastastic breast cancer. J Clin Oncol 2004; 22: 2942–53.

30. McKillop JH. Bone scanning in clinical practice. Springer, Berlin, Heidelberg, New York, 1987, S. 41–57.

31. Gratz S, Becker W. Nuklearmedizinische Untersuchungsmöglichkeiten bei Erkrankungen des Skelettsystems. Radiologe 2000; 40: 953–62.

32. Moser E. Knochenmetastasen – nukleramedizinsche Diagnostik. Skelett-, Knochenmarkszintigraphie oder spezifische Verfahren. Krankenhaus Arzt 1997; 70: 435–9.

33. Creutzig H. Staging of patients with carcinoma of the breast by bone scans? Radiologe 1978; 185: 179–83.

34. Schirrmeister H, Guhlmann A, Kotzerke J et al. Early detection and accurate description of extent of metastatic bone disease in breast cancer with fluoride ion and positron emission tomography. J Clin Oncol 1999; 17: 2381–9.

35. Daldrup-Link HE, Franzius C, Link TM Laukamp D, Sciuk J, Jürgens H, Schober O, Rummeny EJ. Whole-body MR imaging for detection of bone metastases in children and young adults: comparison with bone scintigraphy and FDG-PET. AJR Am J Roentgenol 2001; 177: 229–36.

36. Ferlin G, Rubello D, Chierichetti F, Zanco P, Bergamin R, Trento P, Fin Cargnel S. The role of fluorine-18-deoxyglucose (FDG) positron emission tomography whole body scan (WBS) in staging and follow-up of cancer patients: our first experience. Tumori 1997; 83: 679–84.

37. Kao CH, Hsieh JF, Tsai SC, Ho YJ, Yen RF. Comparison and discrepancy of 18F-2-deoxyglucose positron emission tomography and Tc-99m MDP bone scan to detect bone metastases. Anticancer Res 2000; 20: 2189–92.

38. Franzius C, Daldrup-Link HE, Wagner-Bohn A, Sciuk J, Heindel WL, Jürgens H, Schober O. FDG-PET for detection of recurrences from malignant primary bone tumors comparison with conventional imaging. Annals of Oncology 2002; 13: 157–60.

39. Shreve PD, Barton GH, Gross MD, Wahl RL. Metastatic prostate cancer: Initial findings of PET with 2-Deoxy-2-(F-18)fluoro-d1-glucose. Radiology 1996; 199: 751–6.

40. Chung JK, So Y, Lee JS et al. Value of FDG-PET in papillary thyroid carcinoma with negative 131 I whole-body scan. J Nucl Med 1999; 40: 986–92.

41. Layer G, Sommer T, Busch M, Schüller H, Schild HH. Quantitative Evaluierung der Eignung von Magnetresonanzsequenzen zum Nachweis von Wirbelsäulenmetastasen solider Tumoren. Fortschr Röntgenstr 1998; 168: 20–6.

42. Uhl M, Altehoefer C, Allmann KH, Laubenberger J, Langer M. Radiologische Diagnostik von Knochenmetastasen: Neue Entwicklungen in der Computer- und Magnetresonanztomographie. Krankenhaus Arzt 1997; 70: 430–4.

43. Winterer JT, Ghanem N, Uhl M, Langer M. Radiologische Diagnostik. Skelettäre Metastasen und extraossäre Tumorausdehnung differentialdiagnostisch beurteilen. Klinikarzt 2000; 29: 281–4.

44. Ghanem N, Altehoefer C, Högerle S, Schäfer O, Winterer J, Moser E, Langer M. Comparative diagnostic value and therapeutic relevance of magnetic resonance imaging and bone marrow scintigraphy in patients with metastatic solid tumors of the axial skeleton. Eur J Radiol 2002; 43: 256–61.

45. Vahlensieck M, Layer G. Knochenmark In: MRT des Bewegungsapparats Thieme-Verlag 1997, S. 289–311.

46. Altehoefer C, Bertz H, Ghanem N, Langer M. Extent and time course of morphological changes of bone marrow induced by granulocyte-colony stimulating factor as assessed magnetic resonance imaging of healthy blood stem cell donors. J Magn Reson Imaging 2001; 14: 141–6.

47. Layer G, Sander W, Träber F et al. Diagnostic problems of MRI in studying the effect of G-CSF therapy in bone marrow of patients with malignoma. Radiologe 2000; 40: 710–5.

48. Petren-Mallmin M, Andreasson, Nyman R, et al. Detection of breast cancer metastases in the cervical spine. Acta Radiol 1993; 34: 543–8.

49. Herneth AM, Dominikus M, Kurtaran A, Lang S, Rand T, Kainberger F. Skelettmetastasen: Neue Trends in der bildgebenden Diagnostik. Wien Med Wochenschr Suppl 2002; 113: 92–4.

50. Layer G, Rieker O, Dörr D, Schnakenberg D, Steudel A, Reiser M. MRT und Knochenmarksszintigraphie im Screening von Skelettmetastasen bei Patientinnen mit Mammakarzinom. Fortschr Röntgenstr 1994; 160: 448–52.

51. Daffner RH, Lupetin AR, Dash N, Deeb ZL, Sefczek RJ, Schapiro RL. MRI in the detection of bone marrow. AJR Am J Roentgenol 1986; 146: 353–8.

52. Algra PR, Bloem JL, Tissing H, Falke TH, Arndt JW, Verboom LJ. Detection of vertebral metastases: Comparison between MR imaging and bone scintigraphy. RadioGraphics 1991; 11: 219–32.

53. Avrahami E, Tadmor R, Dally O, Hadar H. Early demonstration of spinal metastases in patients with radiographs and radionuclide bone scans. J Comput Assist Tomogr 1989; 13: 598–602.

54. Kattapuram SV, Khuurana JS, Scott JA, El-Khoury GY. Negative scintigraphy with positive magnetic resonance imaging in bone metastases. Skeletal Radiol 1990; 19: 113–6.

55. Taoka T, Mayr NA, Lee HJ, Yuh WTC, Simonson TM, Karim Rezai K, Berbaum KS. Factors influencing visualization of vertebral metastases on MR imaging versus bone scintigraphy. AJR Am J Roentgenol 2001; 176: 1525–30.

56. Ghanem N, Altehoefer C, Högerle S, Brink I, Ghanem-Wiesel C, Winterer J, Moser E, Langer M. MRI and FDG-PET of the axial skeleton in cancer patients. European Society of Musculoskeletal Radiology, IX Annual Meeting, Valencia 2002, S.191–2.

57. O Connell MJ, Hargaden G, Powell T, Eustace SJ. Whole-body Turbo Short Tau inversion recovery MR imaging using a moving tabletop. AJR Am J Roentgenol 2002; 179: 866–9.

58. Schmidt GP, Baur-Melnyk A, Tiling R, Hahn K, Reiser MF. Comparison of high resolution wholebody MRI using parallel imaging and PET-CT. Radiologe 2004; 44: 889–98.

59. Schmidt GP, Schoenberg SO, Reiser MF, Baur-Melnyk A. Whole-body MR imaging of bone marrow. Eur J Radiol 2005; 55: 33–40.

60. Engelhard K, Hollenbach HP, Wohlfart K, Von Imhoff E, Fellner FA. Comparison of whole-body MRI with automatic moving table technique and bone scintigraphy for screening in patients with breast cancer. Eur Radiol 2004; 14: 99–105.

61. Tamada T, Nagai K, Iizuka M, Imai S, Kajihara Y, Yamamoto S, Kurebayashi J, Shimozuma K, Sonoo H, Fukunaga M. Comparison of whole-body MR imaging and bone scintigraphy in the detection of bone metastases from breast cancer. Nippon Igaku Hoshasen Gakkai Zasshi 2000; 60: 249–54.

62. Lauenstein TC, Freudenberg LS, Goehde SC, Ruehm SG, Goyen M, Bosk S, Debatin JF, Barkhausen J. Whole-body MRI using a rolling for detection of bone metastases. Eur Radiol 2002; 12: 2091–9.

63. Lauenstein TC, Goehde SC, Herborn CU, Goyen M, Oberhoff C, Debatin JF, Ruehm SG, Barkhausen J. Whole-body MR imaging: evaluation of patients for metastases. Radiology 2004; 233: 139–48.

64. Schlemmer HPW, Pfannenberg C, Horger M, Wolfarth K, Tomaschko K, Hebart H, Fenchel M, Miller S, Clausen CD. Clinical utility of a novel whole-body MRI system for comprehensive oncologic staging 11th Proc. Intl. Soc. Magn. Reson. Med., Toronto 2004; 12: 2379.

65. Tausig A, Manthey N, Berger F, Sommer H, Pfluger T, Hahn K. Vorzüge und Limitationen der Ganzkörper-Knochenmark-MRT mit Turbo-STIR-Sequenzen im Vergleich zur planaren Skelettszintigraphie. Nuklearmedizin 2000; 39: 174–9.

66. Schlemmer HP, Schäfer J, Pfannenberg C et al. Fast whole-body assessment of metastatic disease using a novel magnetic resonance imaging system. Initial experiences. Invest Radiol 2005; 40: 64–71.

67. Ghanem N, Bley T, Kelly T, Lohrmann C, Pache G, Saueressig U, Schäfer O, Langer M. Detektion von Knochenmarkmetastasierung und -infiltration in der Ganzkörper-MRT unter Verwendung einer Turbo-STIR-Bildgebung . Fortschr Röntgenstr 2005; 177: 161.

68. Ghanem N, Uhl M, Brink I, Schäfer O, Kelly T, Moser E, Langer M. Diagnostic value of MRI in comparison to scintigraphy, PET, MSCT and PET/CT for the detection of metastases of bone. Eur J Radiol 2005; 55: 41–55.

69. Ghanem N, Schäfer O, Kelly T, Moser E, Langer M. Whole-body MRI in comparison to bone scintigraphy and FDG-PET in detection of bone metastases in patients with solid tumors. MR 2005 MRI – the NOBEL art of imaging with unlimited potential. MR 2005 Garmisch 11th International MRI Symposium 2005, S. 69–70.

70. Laffan EE, O Connor R, Ryan SP, Donoghue VB. Whole-body magnetic resonance imaging: a useful additional sequence in paediatric imaging. Pediatr Radiol 2004; 34: 472–80.

71. Goo HW, Choi SH, Ghim T, Moon HN, Seo JJ. Whole-body MRI of paediatric malignant tumors: comparison with conventional oncological imaging methods. Pediatr Radiol 2005; 35: 792–8.

72. Ghanem NA, Kelly T, Bley TA, Saueressig U, Brink I, Pache G, Langer M. Whole-body MRI in staging cancer patients: a comparison with whole body FDG-PET. 105th Annual Meeting ARRS, May 15–20, 2005, AJR Am J Roentgenol (Suppl) 2005; 184: 41.

73. Mentzel HJ, Kentouche K, Sauner D et al. Comparison of whole-body STIR-MRI and 99mTc-methylene-diphosphonate scintigraphy in children with suspected multifocal bone lesions. Eur Radiol 2004; 14: 2297–2302.

74. Kellenberger CJ, Miller SF, Khan M, Gilday DL, Weitzman S, Babyn PS. Initial experience with FSE STIR whole-body MR imaging for staging lymphoma in children. Eur Radiol 2004; 14: 1829–41.

7 VIBE whole-body MRI for metastasis screening

Thomas C. Lauenstein

7.1 Background

Various whole-body MRI concepts for screening or staging purposes in tumor patients have been presented in the past. Why these whole-body MRI methods have failed to make an impact in clinical routine work is mainly attributable to the following two reasons. First, the investment in time for data acquisition for some examination protocols was far too long [1]. And second, other less time-consuming approaches, especially those using EPI sequences, only offer limited spatial resolution and therefore restricted diagnostic accuracy [2].

It was possible to overcome these limitations with VIBE imaging (volumetric interpolated breath-hold examination). In this type of MR imaging, a T1-weighted, three-dimensional (3D) gradient-echo sequence is used with integrated fat saturation and almost isotropic spatial resolution. Data acquisition takes place with the breath-holding technique; the 3D data sets can be acquired in around 20 s. The VIBE sequence has become established beyond whole-body imaging, especially in the imaging of the abdominal organs [3, 4] as well as the lungs [5]. A comparable image quality to that of conventional 2D gradient-echo sequences can be achieved. With integrated fat saturation, tumors or metastases are easily identified in the parenchymatic organs following intravenous administration of gadolinium due to their significant contrast agent uptake.

7.2 Examination protocol

The basic requirement for whole-body MRI using VIBE is fast patient repositioning, so that different anatomical regions can be examined in quick succession. Two techniques are suitable here: In recent years, patient tables with automatic or manual movement have come into use that allow a surface coil to remain stationary in the isocenter of the magnet during patient movement, thus ensuring high image quality. Newer MR scanners offer the option of using a large number of different coils simultaneously, so that no coil repositioning is necessary here, either, given the additional automated table movement. It is possible in principle to position the patient in the prone as well as the supine position. The supine position is, however, preferable, as this ensures greater patient comfort and the breath-holding technique is easier.

The acquisition of local scout sequences of all regions to be examined (head – thorax – abdomen – pelvis – thigh) serves to verify that complete imaging of the required regions is performed with later imaging sequences. Here it should be ensured that the subsequently acquired VIBE data sets overlap by approx. 2.5 cm to ensure a diagnosis despite possible aliasing artifacts on the cranial or caudal ends of the 3D data sets. Depending on the patient's size, 5 to 6 individual imaging stations should be planned. Especially for large patients, the caudal anatomical regions (lower leg and knee region) should be imaged in two different stations.

Firstly, intravenous administration of a paramagnetic contrast agent (e.g. gadopentetate dimeglumine, Magnevist®, Schering AG, Berlin, Germany) takes place with a dosage of 0.2 mmol/kg body weight and a flow rate of 3.0 ml/s. The first examination station covers the abdomen with a data set acquired 20 s after administration of the contrast agent in an arterial contrast agent phase. A second acquisition is taken in the same patient position a total of 60 s after administration of the contrast agent in a portal-venous phase. Once this second acquisition has been performed, the patient is moved manually or automatically depending on the system so that the thorax, the pelvis, the lower leg, and the head can then be imaged in an equilibrium phase. Finally, another data set should be taken of the abdomen in a late-venous phase. The entire image acquisition time is therefore between four and five minutes. Data acquisition of the liver in three different contrast agent phases is advantageous, because metastases can be differentiated from benign conditions with a high degree of probability [6]. A summary of the most important sequence parameters may be found in Table 7.1. The examination procedure for the respective regions of the body is presented in Table 7.2.

Table 7.1 Recommended parameters for VIBE imaging

TR [ms]	3.1
TE [ms]	1.2
Flip angle [°]	12
Bandwidth [Hz/pixel]	490
Slab thickness [mm]	312
Partitions	104*
Section thickness [mm]	3
Matrix	$240 \times 512^*$
Pixel size [mm × mm]	0.9×0.7
Acquisition time [s]	22

* with interpolation

Table 7.2 Sequence order for VIBE whole-body MRI

	Region of the body	Contrast agent delay [s]
1	Abdomen	20
2	Abdomen	60
3	Thorax	90
4	Pelvis	120
5	Lower leg	150
5b*	Distal lower leg	180
6	Head	180/210+
7	Abdomen	210/240+

* optional, depending on the body size
+ if data acquisition is carried out in Station 5b

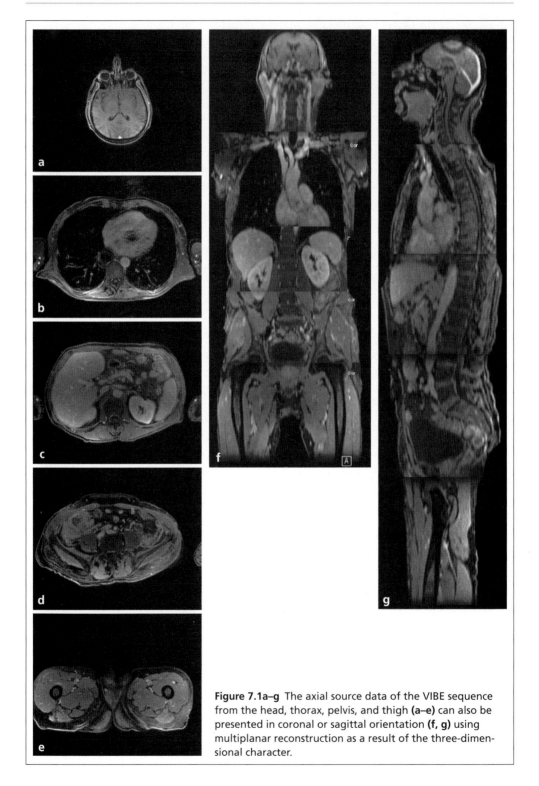

Figure 7.1a–g The axial source data of the VIBE sequence from the head, thorax, pelvis, and thigh **(a–e)** can also be presented in coronal or sagittal orientation **(f, g)** using multiplanar reconstruction as a result of the three-dimensional character.

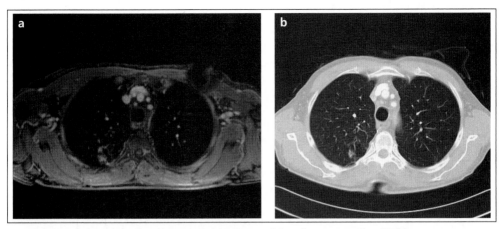

Figure 7.2a, b Lung metastasis detected with VIB-MRI **(a)** and corresponding CT **(b)**.

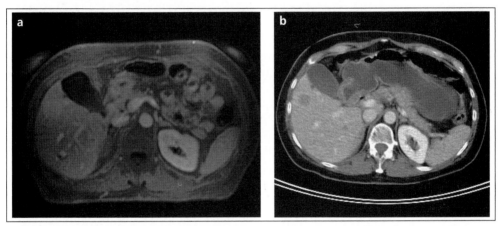

Figure 7.3a, b VIBE imaging shows high sensitivity, especially for the identification of liver metastases **(a)** with good correlation to CT **(b)**.

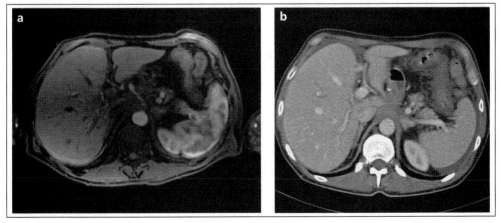

Figure 7.4a, b Adrenal gland metastasis in a patient with bronchial carcinoma identified both in MRI **(a)** as well as CT **(b)**.

Due to the large amount of data and images, the diagnostic viewing should take place at a postprocessing console. As a result of the three-dimensional nature of the VIBE sequence, evaluation in the multiplanar reformation mode (MPR) is desirable so that presentation is also possible in coronal or sagittal orientation, in addition to the axial source images (Fig. 7.1). This evaluation has to take all the relevant organs into consideration, including the head, lungs, liver, adrenal glands, as well as potential stations for lymph node or bone metastases (Figs. 7.2 to 7.4). Information can also be derived on the primary tumor, especially in the case of bronchial carcinoma. Finally, it must be considered that other lesions not directly related with the malignant disease may be detected, especially changes in the arterial vascular system.

7.3   Clinical results

The value of whole-body VIBE MRI has only been described in two clinical studies so far. The first results in a small patient population were presented in 2002 [7]. Four women with identified breast carcinoma and four men with testicular tumors were examined using whole-body VIBE MRI. The number, size, and localization of the identifiable metastases were documented. Reference standards were provided by CT examinations of the head, thorax, abdomen, and pelvis as well as a whole-body bone scintigraphy, which had been performed a few days before the MRI. It was possible to perform whole-body MRI in all eight patients without complications. The average examination time was 11 minutes including positioning of the patient and coils. In this initial feasibility study, whole-body VIBE MRI led to liver metastases being identified in 5 patients and cerebral metastases in 2 patients. The corresponding CT only managed to detect an additional 5 mm lung metastasis. Furthermore, retroperitoneal lymph node metastases were correctly detected in the MRI in one patient and soft tissue metastases in another patient. There were even advantages achieved by MRI compared with bone scintigraphy in the detection of bone metastases. Metastases in the L-spine were found in one patient, which were not detected by bone scintigraphy.

This first feasibility study in general gave rise to further evaluations of the whole-body VIBE concept. The results of a significantly larger patient population were published in 2004 [8]. There were several minor modifications of the examination protocol in this follow-up study. The contrast-enhanced, T1-weighted VIBE data sets were supplemented with fast T2w imaging of the abdomen and thorax. This addition made it possible to classify certain diseases more reliably and in particular to identify fluid accumulations, such as pleural effusion or ascites, without difficulty. 51 patients with various malignant tumors, including breast, bronchial, thyroid and prostrate carcinoma, were studied. Data acquisition took place in the same way as in the first whole-body VIBE study with the aid of a manual movable patient table (Body*SURF*®, MR-Innovation, Essen, Germany, see Chap. 1). Dedicated MRI examinations of the head and individual skeletal sections were used as a standard of reference in this study, as well as the corresponding dedicated CT examinations and bone scintigraphy. The average examination time was less than a quarter of an hour, as in the first study. The data interpretation time was also evaluated, which was 11 minutes on average. Metastases could be ascertained in a total of 43 patients using VIBE MRI, which could be confirmed by reference examinations in 42 patients. Interestingly, for the patient with a discrepant result, a biopsy succeeded in confirming the suspicion of a singular hepatic metastasis so that, in relation to the number of patients, whole-body MRI provided an even higher sensitivity than the previous clinical standard. However, there were clear differences in terms of accuracy of MRI among the various metastasis types. Whereas considerably more liver metastases could be detected by MRI (compared with the corresponding CT), individual lung metastases (<6 mm) were not visible in MRI images. In the group of bone metastases, there were clear differences between scintigraphy and MRI in terms of different anatomical regions: Whereas whole-body scintigraphy was able to detect more lesions in the ribs and the skull, MRI was able to depict more bone metastases in the spinal column and the pelvic region.

The two studies described served to prove the value and, in particular, the clinical practicability of whole-body VIBE MRI. This imaging technique offers reliable tumor staging in less than 15 minutes, and its diagnostic accuracy can even exceed that of the previous clinical routine techniques such as CT or bone scintigraphy in some areas.

7.4   Outlook

The concept of whole-body VIBE MRI holds great potential. Nevertheless, a dedicated MRI examination of an individual region of the body cannot be substituted for by whole-body imaging in the individual case. This means that newer strategies of whole-body MRI integrate a large number of additional MRI sequences in addition to contrast-enhanced VIBE imaging to improve the sensitivity and specificity of MRI [9]. Additional imaging of the head (e.g. with FLAIR sequences) or individual skeletal sections (using STIR sequences) can certainly be helpful. At this juncture, the question should always be asked whether ever-longer examination times as a result of extended sequence protocols really promise additional diagnostic benefit. It is therefore recommended to view VIBE MRI as the basis of a whole-body imaging technique and to expand this individually taking into account the clinically-based tentative diagnoses.

Bibliography

1. Walker R, Kessar P, Blanchard R, et al. Turbo STIR magnetic resonance imaging as a whole-body screening tool for metastases in patients with breast carcinoma: preliminary clinical experience. J Magn Reson Imaging 2000; 11: 343–50.
2. Horvath LJ, Burtness BA, McCarthy S, Johnson KM. Total-body echo-planar MR imaging in the staging of breast cancer: comparison with conventional methods – early experience. Radiology 1999; 211: 119–28.
3. Rofsky NM, Lee VS, Laub G, et al. Abdominal MR imaging with a volumetric interpolated breathhold examination. Radiology 1999; 212: 876–84.
4. Lee VS, Lavelle MT, Rofsky NM, et al. Hepatic MR imaging with a dynamic contrast-enhanced isotropic volumetric interpolated breath-hold examination: feasibility, reproducibility, and technical quality. Radiology 2000; 215: 365–72.
5. Bader TR, Semelka RC, Pedro MS, Armao DM, Brown MA, Molina PL. Magnetic resonance imaging of pulmonary parenchymal disease using a modified breath-hold 3D gradient-echo technique: initial observations. J Magn Reson Imaging 2002; 15: 31–8.

6. Hawighorst H, Schoenberg SO, Knopp MV, Essig M, Miltner P, van Kaick G. Hepatic lesions: morphologic and functional characterization with multiphase breath-hold 3D gadolinium-enhanced MR angiography. Radiology 1999; 210: 89–96.

7. Lauenstein TC, Goehde SC, Herborn CU, et al. Three-dimensional volumetric interpolated breathhold MR imaging for whole-body tumor staging in less than 15 minutes: a feasibility study. AJR Am J Roentgenol. 2002; 179: 445–49.

8. Lauenstein TC, Goehde SC, Herborn CU, et al. Whole-body MR imaging: evaluation of patients for metastases. Radiology 2004; 233: 139–48.

9. Schlemmer HP, Schafer J, Pfannenberg C, et al. Fast whole-body assessment of metastatic disease using a novel magnetic resonance imaging system: initial experiences. Invest Radiol. 2005; 40: 64–71.

8 Whole-body tumor staging: MRI or FDG-PET/CT?

Patrick Veit-Haibach, Andreas Bockisch, Gerald Antoch

8.1 Introduction

The diagnosis and therapy of malignant tumors has become a focus of interest over recent years in the industrial countries as a result of demographic changes. The accurate assessment of the extent of cancerous disease is an essential requirement for efficient therapy, as it is now recognized that the prognosis depends on the stage classification with the application of the appropriate therapy [1–5]. Stage classification of cancerous disease is prescribed by international standards (e.g. American Joint Committee on Cancer, AJCC, or the International Union against Cancer, UICC). This serves to define the stage (TNM stage) based on the size of the primary tumor and any infiltration in the vicinity (T stage), the assessment of metastasis in the local lymph nodes (N stage), and the detection of distant metastases (M stage). Mainly magnetic resonance imaging (MRI), computed tomography (CT), and nuclear medicine techniques, such as positron emission tomography (PET), have become established in the diagnosis of the various tumor types. Besides the absence of radiation exposure, MRI offers the advantage of superior soft tissue contrast and high spatial resolution. The superiority of MRI over CT in the detection of liver and bone lesions has been verified [6, 7]. Whole-body MRI has only been available to a limited extent until recently, however. Disadvantages included long examination times, time-consuming repositioning procedures, and the difficulty of combining several examination sections to form a single image. With the introduction of moving table platform systems and concomitant data acquisition from several surface coils, whole-body MRI has, however, gained continuously in importance. Especially the new and fast sequences have contributed to an improvement in practicability of this examination method in the assessment of the TNM stage [8–11].

In contrast to the predominantly morphological information gained from MRI, PET is a whole-body examination technique which delivers functional information based on the metabolic activity of a tumor. [18F]-2-Fluoro-2-desoxy-D-glucose (FDG) is mainly used as a radioactive pharmaceutical in oncological imaging. FDG is absorbed and metabolized to varying degrees in the different organs depending on their glucose metabolism. Many malignant tumors have a high density of glucose transporters in their cell membranes; they also have an accelerated metabolism due to their malignant growth and therefore show an increased consumption of FDG. On the basis of this functional information, PET demonstrates high accuracy in the detection of malignant tumors, as well as their lymph node metastases, and has already contributed to an improvement in diagnostics for various tumor entities compared with purely morphological imaging techniques [12–14]. However, due to the limited anatomical information provided by PET, a correlation between a morphological technique, such as CT or MRI, is often helpful for precisely locating the tumor. The attempt to retrospectively fuse functional and anatomical data sets has, until now, proven to be complex and not completely reliable and for this reason has not become of widespread importance in clinical routine work, apart from in cerebral imaging.

Since the introduction of combined PET/CT systems, the accurate, co-registered presentation of anatomical and functional image data is now routinely possible [15]. The data sets from both examination techniques are acquired in a single examination procedure and are then precisely fused. As a result of developments in multi-array spiral CT and integration of multi-detector CT systems in PET/CT scanners, fused data sets with CT resolution in the sub-millimeter range with additional metabolic information have become possible. Through the use of combined PET/CT, it has become possible to detect and TNM stage various tumors in oncological imaging with significantly higher precision than with PET or CT alone, as well as in comparison with MRI [16–20]. However, in the literature available to date, there is insufficient information on which indications and cancerous diseases whole-body MRI or whole-body PET/CT is better suited for. For this reason, the current state of scientific knowledge is to be presented at this point and various tumor entities discussed by way of example, where one of the two examination modalities offers advantages over the other.

8.2   Whole-body PET/CT

8.2.1   General technical overview

PET/CT systems from various manufacturers are now commercially available. CT components with 2–64 spiral arrays are currently available. Among the PET detectors, bismuth germanate (BGO), lutetium oxyorthosilicate (LSO) or gadolinium oxyorthosilicate (GSO) are mainly used. The basic approach of combined image acquisition is always founded on the same principle [15] (Fig. 8.1, 8.2).

Firstly the CT is acquired; the duration of the examination essentially depends on the number of detector rows available. The emission data are acquired in PET immediately thereafter. Because the CT data can be used for PET attenuation correction, the acquisition time can be reduced by approx. 30% compared with the PET systems previously available, which required a further transmission measurement for PET attenuation correction. Here the PET examination time depends both on the detector material used and on the activity applied, as well as on the height of the patient, which determines the number of bed positions for the PET. The length of the individual bed positions for PET depends on the device type and can vary between 10 and 15 cm. The scanning time for a bed position is also dependent on the detector material and the patient circumference and typically varies from 3–5 min in everyday clinical work [21]. A total time of 20–40 min therefore needs to be allocated for a PET/CT whole-body examination; reductions in time arise accordingly if only certain parts of the body are examined (Fig. 8.3).

8.2.2   PET/CT acquisition

Several authors exclude the skull in whole-body examinations, as only limited information on cerebral metastases is possible on the basis of the physiological FDG uptake of the brain.

The patients are instructed to abstain from eating for approx. 4–6 h prior to the examination. The blood sugar level, especially of diabetics, should be in the normal range to assure an adequate quality of the examination.

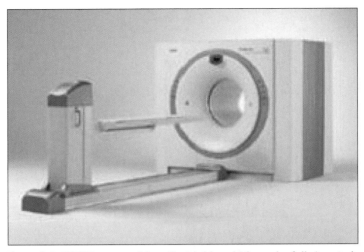

Figure 8.1 PET/CT system with patient table, which can be fully inserted into the system. To prevent deflection of the table, a special device is fixed to the end. The PET/ CT tunnel is longer than for CT or PET on their own, as both scanners have to be accommodated in close proximity to one another (also see Fig. 8.2)

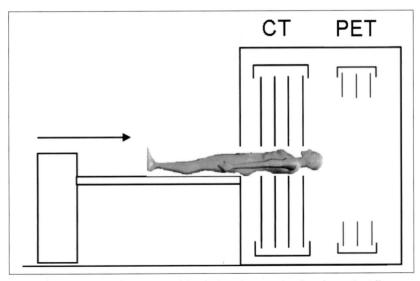

Figure 8.2 Patient on the PET/CT table; during the examination the patient lies on the table in the same position for both of the successive techniques. The CT is firstly acquired in the front part of the system; the detector arrays are only indicated schematically here. The emission data (PET) are captured immediately afterwards in the rear part. The CT data are used for attenuation correction of the positron emission tomography data; PET/CT acquisition is therefore approx. 30% faster than a PET examination.

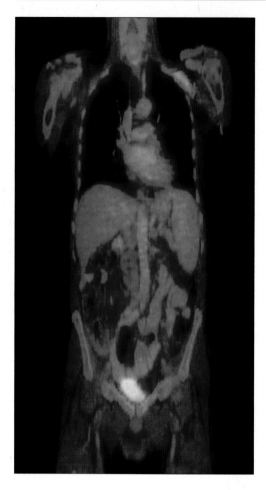

Figure 8.3 Whole-body PET/CT of a patient after resection of a melanoma in the left upper arm. No detection of pathologically increased glucose metabolism. With the combined PET/CT examination, the metabolic PET information is precisely fused with the anatomical CT information over the entire length of the body during data acquisition.

The patients' blood sugar is therefore checked before injecting FDG. The radioactive pharmaceutical FDG is administered intravenously approx. 1 h before the examination. The patients should then sit or lie in a comfortable position to avoid excessive muscular metabolic activation. During this time it is possible for the patient to drink oral contrast agent. Negative oral contrast agent has become established as the substance of choice over positive contrast agents, because an increase in the Hounsfield units from positive contrast agent can cause an artificial increase in the standard uptake value (SUV) – quantification of the FDG uptake in PET – due to the CT-based attenuation correction; thus, artifacts in the PET image can arise. A special negative oral contrast agent consisting of 0.2% carob bean flour and 2.5% mannitol dissolved in 1.5 l water has been found to be suitable in clinical applications so far [22]. Oral contrast agents based on this composition are now commercially available and are in clinical use. The performance of CT examinations can take place with or without intravenous contrast agents dependent on the investigation (see below). The administration and dosage for intravenous contrast agent must be matched to the CT system available (2–64 slices) and corresponds to typical CT protocols.

Typical whole-body PET/CT acquisition parameters are:
- 6–12 bed positions,
- 3–5 min acquisition time per bed position,
- reconstruction with and without attenuation correction to identify potential artifacts.

8.3   Whole-body MRI

8.2.1   General technical overview

Two different systems have been used in practice to date to compare whole-body PET/CT with whole-body MRI: firstly, 32-channel MRI systems are available with which several surface coils (including the head coil) can be positioned simultaneously on the patient. Using the integrated parallel acquisition technique (iPAT), the image data from several of the applied coils can be acquired simultaneously and subsequently reconstructed to form an overall data set (Fig. 8.4). Using this technique, a reduced number of k-space lines is obtained during acquisition. These can then be reconstructed with various algorithms. This takes place either by calculating the missing k-space lines before Fourier transformation (SMASH or GRAPPA) or with the retrospective fusion of the individual images that are obtained (SENSE) [23–25]. The advantages of these acquisition techniques include a high spatial resolution without a significant increase in the acquisition time, or a corresponding reduction in the acquisition time with unchanged resolution. The disadvantage however is the drop in signal-to-noise ratio (SNR). This examination technique has thus far been carried out on a 1.5 Tesla scanner (Magnetom Avanto, Siemens Medical Solutions, Erlangen, Germany). The system can process image information from the connected coil elements on a maximum of 32 channels simultaneously and thus facilitates an examination field of 205 cm with single positioning of the patient (Fig. 8.5).

A further approach for performing a whole-body MRI examination was used in another comparative study [19]. Here a movable table platform for MR scanners is used (Body*SURF*, MR-Innovation, Essen, Germany, see Chap. 1), which allows movement of the patient. Surface coils are used positioned ventrally and dorsally of the patient. The ventrally mounted surface coil is positioned on a device secured to the original patient table so that it can slide over the patient when the patient is moved (Fig. 8.6). The region to be examined is always positioned in the isocenter of the MR scanner. Through the use of parallel image acquisition, high-resolution acquisition from the skull to the feet can be performed with this system.

An examination field of approx. 190 centimeters length is possible with a single positioning of the patient on the mobile part of the table (Fig. 8.7). This system was used with the examinations previously available on a 1.5 Tesla system (Magnetom Sonata®, Siemens Medical Solutions, Erlangen, Germany); this mobile system can, however, in principle be used with other Siemens MR scanners.

8.3.2   MRI examination

Various sequences were used during the examination in axial and coronal orientations with the 32-channel system described (e.g. STIR, HASTE, T1 with and without contrast agent). Here it is important to mention that with contrast-enhanced sequences (3D VIBE),

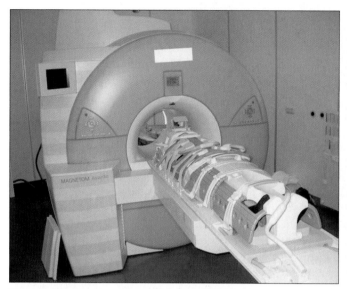

Figure 8.4 Patient in supine, head-first position. The patient is covered with several surface coils. The whole body can therefore be captured using parallel image acquisition in all three planes.

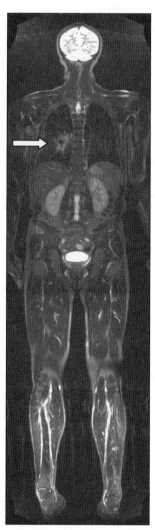

Figure 8.5 Whole-body MRI examination of a patient with a non small-cell bronchial carcinoma (white arrow right half of the thorax). Coronal whole-body image using a STIR sequence.

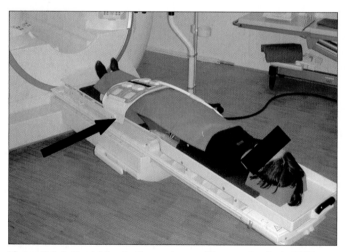

Figure 8.6 Patient lying in the supine position on the Body*SURF* system.
The roller-mounted patient platform is mounted as an accessory on top of the original MRI table and can be moved over the entire length. The integrated surface coil is locked on a device fixated to the original table (black arrow). The patient can be moved under this surface coil, which facilitates axial acquisition of nearly the whole body.

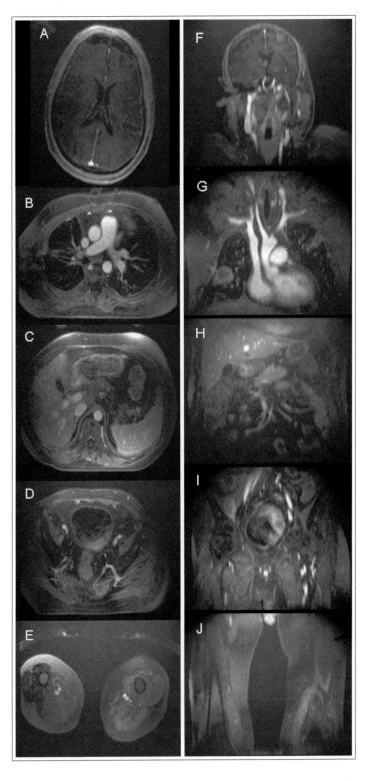

Figure 8.7A–J Axial orientation with the Body*SURF* system to the distal thighs. **(A)** Image of the head (axial) with a contrast-enhanced T1 sequence. **(B)** Image of the thorax (axial) with a contrast-enhanced 3D VIBE sequence. **(C)** Image of the abdomen (axial) with a contrast-enhanced 3D VIBE sequence. **(D)** Image of the pelvis (axial) with a contrast-enhanced 3D VIBE sequence. **(E)** Image of the thighs (axial) with a contrast-enhanced 3D VIBE sequence. All sequences specified were acquired sequentially in a single examination procedure. The patient remained lying on the table in an unchanged position throughout. **(F–J)** Corresponding coronal reconstruction of the axial image stations. Patient with a non small-cell bronchial carcinoma in the right lung **(G)**.

a dynamic examination with early arterial, portal venous and late venous sequences was carried out. The overall acquisition time was approx. 55 min using this system; the sequence protocols should be adapted here dependent on the investigation, however.

A similar sequence order with the corresponding technical parameters was used with the moving table platform. After acquiring the unenhanced sequences from the thorax and upper abdomen, enhanced acquisition can also be performed in this case with contrast agent (3D VIBE) in the dynamic flow phases described above. A single sequence for the specified protocol lasts 22 s. An examination of this type takes approx. 30 min overall. It is possible to extend the sequences without difficulty depending on the relevant indication.

8.4 Previous clinical results

8.4.1 T stage

The T stage firstly specifies the size of the primary tumor and secondly the relationship and extent of the primary tumor with reference to the surrounding organs. As a result of its very good soft tissue contrast, MRI is often superior to CT in this respect. However, as a purely morphological technique, it lacks functional information; this is supplemented by the PET examination. Due to the limited anatomical information provided by PET, a morphological technique should be called upon if at all possible to assess and define the T stage (Fig. 8.8).

The accuracy of whole-body MRI and whole-body FDG-PET/CT in the assessment of the T stage has only been investigated with various tumor entities in one study so far. The T stage was correctly assessed with FDG-PET/CT in 80% of tumors, with MRI in just 52% [19]. Apart from the more accurate assessment of the T stage due to the functional data additionally available in PET, the makeup of the patient collective certainly also had an influence on these results. A large number of patients had a bronchial carcinoma as the underlying disease. FDG-PET/CT is known to be particularly accurate here, whereas the diagnostic accuracy of MRI for lung tumors is still subject to controversial discussion today [26, 27].

8.4.2 N stage

The lymph node stage is another important parameter with respect to staging cancerous disease. Lymph nodes are differentiated morphologically into benign and malignant on the basis of their size. According to experience, however, characterization on the basis of size alone is only possible with limited accuracy. A lymph node can be enlarged due to an inflammatory reaction and not be infiltrated by metastasis. On the other hand, micrometastases may already exist in lymph nodes without pathological enlargement of the lymph node. It has already been demonstrated in the case of various malignant diseases that up to 20% of lymph nodes near tumors and not enlarged are already infiltrated with metastases, whereas up to 40% of lymph nodes exceeding the applicable pathological size criteria are not infiltrated with tumors [28–30]. The sensitivities of purely morphological techniques for lymph node staging lie between 58% and 88%, the specificities between 58% and 86% e.g. for lymph nodes associated with head-neck tumors [31]. Similar sensitivities and specificities are known for the evaluation of abdominal lymph nodes. The CT sensitivities in these cases is stated as up to 40–72% and specificities up to 90%, depending in each case on

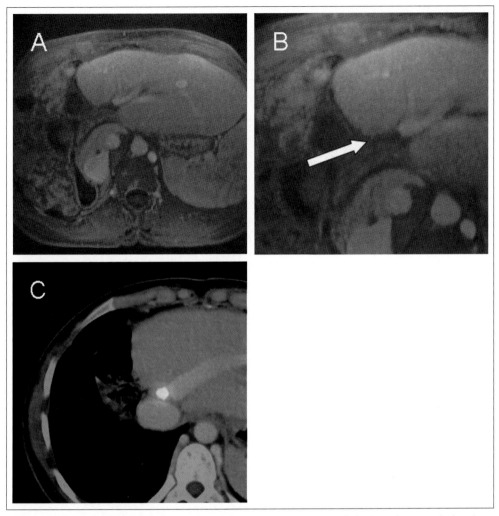

Figure 8.8A–C Female patient after surgery (trisegmental resection) of the liver due to a cholangiocellular carcinoma. Rising tumor marker for approx. 8 months, MRI controls negative. **(A)** Contrast-enhanced MRI of the abdomen (axial 3D VIBE); after hepatic partial resection, parts of the intestine lie next to the hypertrophied left liver lobe. **(B)** Enlargement and focusing on the hepatic veins. A hypodense structure is apparent next to the middle hepatic vein with low marginal CA uptake (white arrow); judged in MRI to be a postoperative residual, non-malignant result. **(C)** Axial, contrast-enhanced FDG-PET/CT: focal increase in glucose utilization of a highly suspicious malignancy lying directly beneath the middle liver vein and adjacent to the inferior vena cava. The female patient had a recurrence in this region.

the patient collective and study design [32, 33]. MRI, as a morphological technique, shows overall comparable values [34].

In this context, PET has shown its superiority over morphological techniques in the assessment of the N stage. The values cited in the literature fluctuate e.g. for staging thoracic and cervical lymph nodes between 87% and 94% for sensitivities, and between 86% and 96% for specificities [32, 35, 36]. For abdominal lymph nodes the values lie between 75% and 91% (sensitivity) and 92% and 100% (specificity) [37]. In direct comparison with PET on its own, PET/CT showed a significantly higher sensitivity in patients with bronchial tumors [35]. Based on this preliminary study, a higher accuracy of PET/CT in the evaluation of the N stage compared with the purely morphological technique of MRI is expected. In comparison of different tumor entities, significantly more accurate evaluation of the N stage is shown with FDG-PET/CT (93%), with a sensitivity of 95% and a specificity of 92%.

MRI showed an accuracy of 79%, a sensitivity of 79%, and a specificity of 78% [19]. Schmidt et al. [38] was largely able to confirm these results by using a 32-channel system with an MRI sensitivity of 83% and a specificity of 85% in correlation with PET/CT as the standard of reference. A direct comparison of the two examination methods in patients with non small-cell bronchial carcinoma also succeeded in proving the significant advantage of PET/CT over MRI [39] (Fig. 8.9). It must still be investigated on an individual basis in which tumor entities this superiority is to be found. There are indications that the sensitivities and specificities in lymph node detection of metastasized melanomas do not differ between MRI and PET/CT [40].

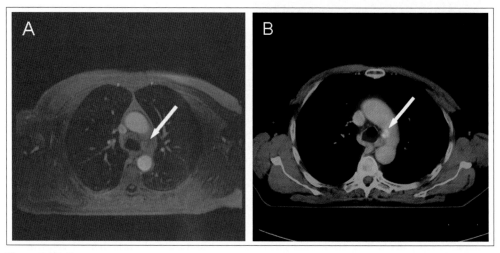

Figure 8.9A, B
(A) Axial, contrast-enhanced MRI image (3D VIBE) in a patient with a non small-cell bronchial carcinoma. A non-pathologically enlarged mediastinal lymph node is apparent (white arrow). MRI judged the lymph node as non-malignant.
(B) Axial, contrast-enhanced FDG-PET/CT: The same patient shows a non-pathologically enlarged mediastinal lymph node with significantly increased glucose utilization. The lymph node was assessed as malignant from the PET/CT. The result was subsequently histopathologically verified with a mediastinoscopy.

8.4.3 M stage

In an evaluation of the M stage, a study from Antoch et al. [19] revealed no significant difference between whole-body PET/CT and whole-body MRI. PET/CT showed sensitivity and specificity of 93% and 95% respectively, as well as an accuracy of 94%, whereas MRI

Figure 8.10A, B
(A) Axial, contrast-enhanced MRI image (3D VIBE) of a female patient with a recurrent mamma carcinoma. Hypodense, irregularly contoured and low CA absorbing lesion in the right-sided pubic ramus (white arrow). MRI assessed the result as bone metastasis.
(B) Axial, contrast-enhanced FDG-PET/CT of the same patient. Focal increased glucose utilization in a bone osteolysis (white arrow); PET/CT also evaluated the result as bone metastasis.

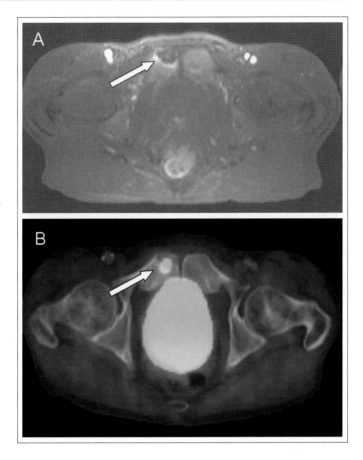

achieved values of 90%, 95%, and 93%. The different organ systems should however be distinguished here: MRI was considerably more sensitive than PET/CT in the detection of bone lesions (85% versus 62%), although the difference in specificity was not significant (92% versus 96%). MRI and PET are discussed controversially in the literature for detection of bone metastases (Fig. 8.10). Some studies consider MR examination to be more accurate, others PET [41–43]. MRI was also superior to FDG-PET/CT in the detection of liver metastases; here the sensitivities and specificities of MRI were 93% and 95%, whereas the PET/CT values attained were 86% and 96% [44]. In the evaluation of metastasis of the lung, PET/CT was, on the other hand, more accurate than MRI. Schmidt et al. state the sensitivity, specificity, and accuracy of MRI in the detection of distant metastases as 91%, 87%, and 90% compared with PET/CT as the standard of reference.

8.5 Summary and outlook

With combined whole-body PET/CT and whole-body MRI, two methods are available which are in a position to replace the previous multimodal staging strategies in oncological diagnostics [17–19, 38, 45, 46]. Concepts for oncological whole-body imaging are not new, but whole-body MRI and also whole-body PET were very time-consuming until a few years ago, and, at least in the case of MRI, routine clinical application was only possible to a very limited extent. The use of whole-body MRI has received an enormous impetus through recent technological developments [9, 10, 11, 47]. With the development of faster sequences, movable table platforms, multi-channel technology, and multiplanar reconstruction options, whole-body MRI has now moved into the focus of clinical applications.

As a result of the CT-based attenuation correction, it is possible with PET/CT to reduce the examination time by approx. 30–40% compared with PET and, at the same time, to obtain a hitherto unique combination of morphological and metabolic information in a single examination procedure.

8.5.1   Indications for FDG-PET/CT and MRI

As previously mentioned, there are still only two studies available comparing combined whole-body PET/CT and whole-body MRI. These both involved investigating an inhomogeneous patient population with various tumor entities. The decision in favor of whole-body MRI or whole-body PET/CT is essentially influenced by the tumor entity studied. As FDG has primarily been used so far as the radioactive agent in combined PET/CT, an advantage of PET/CT over MRI is only to be expected with FDG-PET-positive tumors. Only then can the additional metabolic information from PET/CT be used to improve the diagnosis. Various tumors show no increased glucose utilization and are therefore only of limited suitability for a PET/CT examination. For instance, according to the literature currently available, only between 0 and 64% of primary hepatocellular carcinomas (HCC) are PET-positive [48, 49]. Our own experience shows that HCC is FDG-PET-positive in approx. 40% of cases. Limited sensitivities are also known for FDG-PET imaging with carcinomas of the gastrointestinal tract [50]. New and alternative tracers, such as DOTATOC, promise improved diagnostic efficacy in this field. Many neuroendocrine tumors of the pancreas, medullary thyroid carcinomas, pheochromocytomas, and Merkel cell tumors are therefore also not typical indications for FDG-PET/CT [51]. For prostate and bladder carcinomas, as well as for renal cell carcinoma, there is also only a low PET positivity to be expected; here, superiority of MRI over FDG-PET/CT imaging is to be anticipated. Especially for prostate carcinoma, however, another tracer (choline) has become established as an alternative to FDG.

But even in the case of PET positivity of lymph node and distant metastases, MRI can yield results of an equivalent quality to those from FDG-PET/CT. Our own experience with melanoma patients shows comparable sensitivities of MRI and PET/CT in the detection of lymph node metastases. This is also attributable to the fact that melanomas with a certain tumor depth cause primary lymphogenous micrometastasis. These micrometastases can be detected neither with MRI nor with PET/CT on account of their small size. It remains to be seen which of the two modalities can first detect a recurrent tumor based on occult metastasis. Common FDG-PET-positive tumors are thyroid carcinoma, head-neck tumors, esophagus carcinomas, colorectal carcinomas, mamma and ovarian carcinomas, lymphomas, melanomas, and lung tumors.

It has been possible to prove the superiority of FDG-PET/CT over whole-body MRI in staging and influencing the therapy regime of various tumor entities. However, a differentiated view cannot help identifying that MRI appears superior in the detection of bone and liver lesions. This may to some extent be because the liver lesions in the available studies were often smaller than 1 cm. As the acquisition of PET/CT takes approx. 3–5 min per bed position with shallow breathing, the breathing displacement of the liver can cause a blurring effect on the image and the increased FDG uptake can be „smeared" in the image. The increased glucose utilization is no longer identifiable, and a lesion cannot be detected or is erroneously evaluated as benign.

In the detection of bone metastases, the superiority of MRI for a PET-negative primary tumor is easy to explain. But PET also appears to be insensitive compared with MRI in the detection of diffuse, non-focal bone marrow metastasis. In MRI such cases have been diagnosed as true positive as a result of the bone marrow edema, as well as the diffuse increase in contrast agent uptake. The resolving power of the PET components (approx. 4–5 mm) can also be an important reason for the absence of detection of small lesions. It also remains to be seen here whether an advancement of PET/CT systems through an improvement in resolution will affect the accuracy of tumor staging.

In contrast, PET/CT appears to be superior to MRI in the detection of lung metastases. This superiority is primarily based on the high sensitivity of CT in the detection of lung metastases. As in the case of the liver, PET can miss small lesions owing to the blurring effect. Following the introduction of fast pulse sequences, a few studies have verified similar detection rates for lung lesions for both MRI and spiral CT. Further studies dedicated to this question are expected.

Whole-body FDG-PET/CT was superior to MRI in lymph node diagnostics with various tumor entities. However, through the use of ultra-small superparamagnetic iron oxide (USPIO) contrast agents, MRI shows a significant improvement in lymph node diagnostics. Clinical applications associated with whole-body MRI or in comparison with PET/CT are not yet available, though.

Systematic differences arise between the various MRI protocols. While the study from Antoch et al. stated a time requirement of approx. 35 min for whole-body MRI, the protocol from Schmidt et al. required approx. 55 min. The essential difference was that in the first study the FOV (field of view) did not cover the lower legs. These could also have been imaged with the moving table platform system; however, this would have necessitated repositioning the patients and thereby substantially prolonged the examination time. As all the lymphatic drainage pathways, all abdominal organs, and the axial skeleton were included in the examination, this additional effort did not seem to be justified to the authors. An essential advantage of the whole-body MRI protocols compared with PET/CT is, however, the inclusion of the brain in the examination procedure, as cerebral metastases have an essential impact on the prognosis and consequently on the patient's therapy regime. Although the head can also be studied with FDG-PET/CT, the sensitivity of FDG for small cerebral lesions is low on account of the physiologically intense glucose utilization of the brain. Optimization of the CT acquisition could bring about an improvement in the sensitivity of PET/CT, but, as is known from comparisons of CT with MRI, the sensitivities of MRI will not be attained.

Additional disadvantages of whole-body PET/CT are the not insignificant radiation doses to the patient, which amounts to approx. 22 mSv for an examination from the head to the thighs. Of this, approx. 7 mSv are attributable to the PET and approx. 15 mSv to the CT if a diagnostic CT is acquired. In the view of the authors, a diagnostic CT component is indispensable to be able to anatomically classify increased glucose utilization of PET accurately and, if required, to have the CT data available for a diagnosis in the case of a FDG-

PET-negative lesion. The response of the tumor is evaluated in follow-up examinations under therapy based on the intensity of the tracer uptake, so that in these cases a low dose component appears sufficient for clinical monitoring.

Last but not least, today the choice of technique is also decided by the availability of equipment. Combined PET/CT systems are only installed in a few centers in Germany, but are becoming increasingly widespread internationally. The further spread of PET/CT is currently hindered in Germany by the failure of the statutory health insurance to cover the costs of the examination. Whole-body MRI systems, on the other hand, are increasingly available, and their number exceeds that of PET/CT systems many times over. The question as to whether a PET/CT or MRI is performed ultimately has to be made dependent on availability and the tumor entity.

Bibliography

1. Kanellos I. Progress in the treatment of colorectal cancer. Tech Coloproctol 2004 Nov; 8 (Suppl 1): 1–2.
2. O'Connell JB, Maggard MA, Ko CY. Colon cancer survival rates with the new American Joint Committee on Cancer sixth edition staging. J Natl Cancer Inst 2004; 96(19): 1420–5.
3. Cerny T, Giaccone G. Pleura mesothelioma: combined modality treatments. Ann Oncol 2002; 13 (Suppl 4): 217–25.
4. Cerny T, Gillessen S. Advances in the treatment of non-Hodgkin's lymphoma. Ann Oncol 2002; 13 (Suppl 4): 211–6.
5. AJCC. AJCC Cancer Staging Manual, Sixth Edition: Springer, 2002.
6. Semelka RC, Martin DR, Balci C, Lance T. Focal liver lesions: comparison of dual-phase CT and multisequence multiplanar MR imaging including dynamic gadolinium enhancement. J Magn Reson Imaging 2001; 13: 397–401.
7. Semelka RC, Worawattanakul S, Kelekis NL, John G, Woosley JT, Graham M, Cance WG. Liver lesion detection, characterization, and effect on patient management: comparison of single-phase spiral CT and current MR techniques. J Magn Reson Imaging 1997; 7(6): 1040–7.
8. Lauenstein TC, Freudenberg LS, Goehde SC, et al. Whole-body MRI using a rolling table platform for the detection of bone metastases. Eur Radiol 2002; 12: 2091–9.
9. Barkhausen J, Quick HH, Lauenstein T, et al. Whole-body MR imaging in 30 seconds with real-time true FISP and a continuously rolling table platform: feasibility study. Radiology 2001; 220: 252–6.
10. Goehde SC, Hunold P, Vogt FM, Ajaj W, Goyen M, Herborn CU, Forsting M, Debatin JF, Ruehm SG. Full-body cardiovascular and tumor MRI for early detection of disease: feasibility and initial experience in 298 subjects. AJR Am J Roentgenol 2005; 184(2): 598–611.
11. Lauenstein TC, Goehde SC, Herborn CU, Goyen M, Oberhoff C, Debatin JF, Ruehm SG, Barkhausen J. Whole-body MR imaging: evaluation of patients for metastases. Radiology. 2004; 233(1): 139–48.
12. Haberkorn U, Schoenberg SO. Imaging of lung cancer with CT, MRT and PET. Lung Cancer 2001; 34 (Suppl 3): 13–23.
13. Kinkel K, Lu Y, Both M, Warren RS, Thoeni RF. Detection of hepatic metastases from cancers of the gastrointestinal tract by using noninvasive imaging methods (US, CT, MR imaging, PET): a metaanalysis. Radiology 2002; 224(3): 748–56.
14. Kantorova I, Lipska L, Belohlavek O, Visokai V, Trubac M, Schneiderova M. Routine (18)F-FDG PET preoperative staging of colorectal cancer: comparison with conventional staging and its impact on treatment decision making. J Nucl Med 2003; 44: 1784–8.

15. Beyer T, Townsend DW, Brun T, et al. A combined PET/CT scanner for clinical oncology. J Nucl Med 2000; 41: 1369–79.
16. Delbeke D, Martin WH. PET and PET-CT for evaluation of colorectal carcinoma. Semin Nucl Med 2004; 34: 209–23.
17. Veit P, Antoch G, Bockisch A, Ruehm S. Dual-modality PET/CT and lymph node detection: enhancing the diagnostic accuracy in oncologic staging. Eur Radiol 2005; in press
18. Antoch G, Saoudi N, Kuehl H, Dahmen G, Mueller SP, Beyer T, Bockisch A, Debatin JF, Freudenberg LS. Accuracy of whole-body dual-modality fluorine-18-2-fluoro-2-deoxy-D-glucose positron emission tomography and computed tomography (FDG-PET/CT) for tumor staging in solid tumors: comparison with CT and PET. J Clin Oncol 2004; 22(21): 4357–68.
19. Antoch G, Vogt FM, Freudenberg LS, Nazaradeh F, Goehde SC, Barkhausen J, Dahmen G, Bockisch A, Debatin JF, Ruehm SG. Whole-body dual-modality PET/CT and whole-body MRI for tumor staging in oncology. JAMA 2003; 290(24): 3199–206.
20. Schmidt GP, Schmid R, Hahn K, Reiser MF. Whole-body MRI and PET/CT in tumor diagnosis. Radiologe 2004; 44(11): 1079–87.
21. Halpern BS, Dahlbom M, Quon A, et al. Impact of patient weight and emission scan duration on PET/CT image quality and lesion detectability. J Nucl Med 2004; 45: 797–801.
22. Antoch G, Kuehl H, Kanja J, Lauenstein TC, Schneemann H, Hauth E, Jentzen W, Beyer T, Goehde SC, Debatin JF. Dual-modality PET/CT scanning with negative oral contrast agent to avoid artifacts: introduction and evaluation. Radiology 2004; 230(3): 879–85.
23. Pruessmann KP, Weiger M, Scheidegger MB, Boesiger P. SENSE: sensitivity encoding for fast MRI. Magn Reson Med 1999; 42(5): 952–62.
24. Sodickson DK, Griswold MA, Jakob PM. SMASH imaging. Magn Reson Imaging Clin N Am 1999; 7(2): 237–54.
25. Griswold MA, Jakob PM, Heidemann RM, Nittka M, Jellus V, Wang J, Kiefer B, Haase A. Generalized autocalibrating partially parallel acquisitions (GRAPPA). Magn Reson Med 2002; 47(6): 1202–10.
26. Beets-Tan RG, Beets GL. Rectal cancer: review with emphasis on MR imaging. Radiology 2004; 232(2): 335–46.
27. Gdeedo A, Van Schil P, Corthouts B, Van Mieghem F, Van Meerbeeck J, Van Marck E. Comparison of imaging TNM [(i)TNM] and pathological TNM [pTNM] in staging of bronchogenic carcinoma. Eur J Cardiothorac Surg 1997; 12(2): 224–7.
28. Deslauriers J, Gregoire J. Clinical and surgical staging of non-small cell lung cancer. Chest 2000; 117 (4 Suppl 1): 96S–103S.
29. Staples CA, Muller NL, Miller RR, Evans KG, Nelems B. Mediastinal nodes in bronchogenic carcinoma: comparison between CT and mediastinoscopy. Radiology 1988; 167(2): 367–72.
30. Dwamena BA, Sonnad SS, Angobaldo JO, Wahl RL. Metastases from non-small cell lung cancer: mediastinal staging in the 1990s – meta-analytic comparison of PET and CT. Radiology 1999; 213: 530–6.
31. Schoder H, Yeung HW. Positron emission imaging of head and neck cancer, including thyroid carcinoma. Semin Nucl Med 2004; 34: 180–97.
32. Torabi M, Aquino SL, Harisinghani MG. Current concepts in lymph node imaging. J Nucl Med 2004; 45: 1509–18.
33. Gretschel S, Moesta KT, Hunerbein M, et al. New concepts of staging in gastrointestinal tumors as a basis of diagnosis and multimodal therapy. Onkologie 2004; 27: 23–30.
34. Thoeni RF. Colorectal cancer. Radiologic staging. Radiol Clin North Am 1997; 35: 457–85.
35. Antoch G, Stattaus J, Nemat AT, et al. Non-small cell lung cancer: dual-modality PET/CT in preoperative staging. Radiology 2003; 229: 526–33.
36. Rieber A, Schirrmeister H, Gabelmann A, et al. Pre-operative staging of invasive breast cancer with MR mammography and/or PET: boon or bunk? Br J Radiol 2002; 75: 789–98.
37. Follen M, Levenback CF, Iyer RB, et al. Imaging in cervical cancer. Cancer 2003; 98: 2028–38.

38. Schmidt GP, Baur-Melnyk A, Tiling R, et al. Comparison of high resolution whole-body MRI using parallel imaging and PET-CT. First experiences with a 32-channel MRI system. Radiologe 2004, 44(9): 889–98.

39. Veit P, Vogt FM, Freudenberng L, et al. Comparison of whole-body PET/CT and whole-body MRI in patients with newly diagnosed NSCLC. Abstractbook, RSNA-Meeting Chicago, Nov. 2004, p. 383.

40. Vogt FM, Veit P, Jablonka R, Massing S, Ruehm S, Antoch G. Whole-body MRI versus whole-body PET/CT in staging of newly diagnosed malignangt melanoma: initial results. Abstractbook, RSNA-Meeting Chicago, Nov. 2004, p. 371.

41. Daldrup-Link HE, Franzius C, Link TM, Laukamp D, Sciuk J, Jurgens H, Schober O, Rummeny EJ. Whole-body MR imaging for detection of bone metastases in children and young adults: comparison with bone scintigraphy and FDG PET. AJR Am J Roentgenol 2001; 177(1): 229–36.

42. Franzius C, Daldrup-Link HE, Wagner-Bohn A, Sciuk J, Heindel WL, Jurgens H, Schober O. FDG-PET for detection of recurrences from malignant primary bone tumors: comparison with conventional imaging. Ann Oncol 2002; 13(1): 157–60.

43. Nakamoto Y, Osman M, Wahl RL. Prevalence and patterns of bone metastases detected with positron emission tomography using F-18 FDG. Clin Nucl Med, 2003, 28(4): 302–7.

44. Kinkel K, Lu Y, Both M, Warren RS, Thoeni RF. Detection of hepatic metastases from cancers of the gastrointestinal tract by using noninvasive imaging methods (US, CT, MR imaging, PET): a metaanalysis. Radiology 2002; 224(3): 748–56.

45. Lardinois D, Weder W, Hany TF, et al. Staging of non-small-cell lung cancer with integrated positron-emission tomography and computed tomography. N Engl J Med 2003; 348(25): 2500–7.

46. Veit P, Kuehle C, Beyer T, et al. Whole-body PET/CT tumor staging with integrated PET/CT-colonography: technical feasibility and first experiences in patients with colorectal cancer. GUT 2005; in press.

47. Goyen M, Quick HH, Debatin JF, et al. Whole-body three-dimensional MR angiography with a rolling table platform: initial clinical experience. Radiology Jul 2002; 224(1): 270–7.

48. Teefey SA, Hildeboldt CC, Dehdashti F, Siegel BA, Peters MG, Heiken JP, Brown JJ, McFarland EG, Middleton WD, Balfe DM, Ritter JH. Detection of primary hepatic malignancy in liver transplant candidates: prospective comparison of CT, MR imaging, US, and PET. Radiology 2003; 226(2): 533–42.

49. Wudel LJ Jr, Delbeke D, Morris D, Rice M, Washington MK, Shyr Y, Pinson CW, Chapman WC. The role of [18F]fluorodeoxyglucose positron emission tomography imaging in the evaluation of hepatocellular carcinoma. Am Surg 2003; 69(2): 117–24.

50. Adams S, Baum R, Rink T, Schumm-Drager PM, Usadel KH, Hor G. Limited value of fluorine-18 fluorodeoxyglucose positron emission tomography for the imaging of neuroendocrine tumors. Eur J Nucl Med 1998; 25(1): 79–83.

51. Reske SN, Kotzerke J. FDG-PET for clinical use. Results of the 3rd German Interdisciplinary Consensus Conference, „Onko-PET III", 21 July and 19 September 2000. Eur J Nucl Med 2001; 28(11): 1707–23.

52. Vogt FM, Herborn CU, Hunold P, et al. HASTE MRI versus chest radiography in the detection of pulmonary nodules: comparison with MDCT. AJR Am J Roentgenol 2004; 183(1): p 71–8.

53. Clement O, Luciani A. Imaging the lymphatic system: possibilities and clinical applications. Eur Radiol 2004; 14(8): 1498–507.

9　Whole-body tumor staging with specific contrast agents

Alexander Huppertz

Organ-specific MRI contrast agents have been intensively developed since the early 1980s to change the signal properties in defined target organs such that immigrant pathological tissue can be reliably distinguished.

Besides the liver, other organs can be studied with specific contrast agents injectable in bolus form, so that the use of whole-body MRI opens up expanded options in tumor staging. In the case of the iron-oxide-based lymph node specific contrast agents, coverage of the whole body is often necessary to be in a position to evaluate the lymph drainage pathways over long distances.

9.1　Liver-specific contrast agents

The liver-specific MRI contrast agents can be classified into two groups: firstly the super-paramagnetic iron oxides (SPIO), which lead to a signal drop in the healthy hepatic parenchyma in T2-weighted images (healthy liver becomes black), and secondly paramagnetic contrast agents, which effect a signal increase of the healthy hepatic parenchyma in T1-weighted images (healthy liver becomes white).

For whole-body imaging, only the paramagnetic T1 contrast agents Primovist® (gadoxetic acid, Schering AG, Berlin, Germany) and MultiHance® (gadobenate dimeglumine, Altanapharma, Konstanz, Germany) can be used. Both contrast agents show the well-known contrast effects shortly after injection in the arterial and venous perfusion phases for unspecific, extracellular contrast agents (e.g. Magnevist®, Schering AG, Berlin, Germany).

Primovist® has a higher liver specificity and therefore provides the most favorable conditions for the detection of liver metastases. Roughly 50% of the administered dose is absorbed by the liver [1]. A European multicenter study showed that Primovist® allows significantly improved detection and localization of liver lesions [2]. In particular, small lesions under 10 mm in diameter are more reliably discovered. The characterization of the lesions discovered is also improved [2–3].

Both the good detection of focal lesions [4] and the higher extracellular T1 effect speak in favor of the use of MultiHance®, as the contrast agent is administered in higher doses compared with Primovist® (at least 0.05 mmol/kg body weight for MultiHance® compared with 0.025 mmol/kg body weight for Primovist® with comparable relaxivity). A disadvantage however is the longer period of time before acquisition of the liver-specific images (40–120 min after application).

9.2 Whole-body MRI with liver-specific contrast agents in patients with rectal carcinoma

A rectosigmoidoscopy or colonoscopy with biopsy is recommended for staging a rectal carcinoma. Endosonography should also be performed. In terms of imaging diagnostics, an X-ray examination of the lungs in two planes or a thorax CT and a computed tomography (CT) of the abdomen is recommended [5]. Current studies have shown that thin-slice MRI of the rectum shows high accuracy for TN staging [6–7]. Following the results of an extensive multicenter study, it was recently recommended to routinely include MRI in the staging concept for rectal carcinoma [7–8]. According to current knowledge, this exclusively involves the use of thin-slice T2-weighted sequences in axial and sagittal orientation [9–10]; an additional evaluation of T1-weighted sequences after administration of extracellular gadolinium-based contrast agents showed no increase in the diagnostic accuracy [11]. In up to 30% of patients with identified rectal carcinoma, liver metastases already exist at the time of the first diagnosis. The liver represents by far the most frequent localization of hematogenous metastasis (approx. 75%). The second most frequent site of metastasis is the lung (approx. 15%); the skeletal system and the neurocranium are only rarely affected.

This constellation, i.e. a high prevalence of liver metastasis at the time of the primary diagnosis, a change in the therapeutic strategy in the case of diagnosis of liver lesions, and the lack of necessity for contrast-enhanced dynamics in staging the primary tumor, represent the ideal conditions for the use of liver-specific contrast agents for full TNM staging. The aim of this approach is to combine the currently highest accuracy for the detection of liver metastases [2], precise diagnostics of pulmonary [12] and abdominal metastases, and an unaltered accuracy for TN staging of the primary tumor into a single examination.

The examination with a whole-body MR scanner with TIM (Total Imaging Matrix) technology (Magnetom Avanto, Siemens Medical Solutions, Erlangen, Germany) includes the depiction of the rectum, liver, lung, abdomen, and pelvis (Table 9.1). Matrix coils are used (24-channel spine coil and two to three 6-channel body coils depending on the size of patient). The sequences used for rectum, liver, and lung are summarized in Tables 9.2–9.4.

The examination starts with the thin-slice imaging of the rectum in axial and sagittal orientation (Fig. 9.1). T2-weighted sequences are used exclusively.

The liver is then imaged unenhanced with T1-weighting. Administration of Primovist® then follows as a fast injection at 1–2 ml/s; the arterial phase (approx. 15 s after injection) and the portal-venous phase (approx. 50 s after injection) of the liver are acquired with a 3D sequence. Immediately thereafter, the lung is imaged in the venous phase, also with the use of a 3D se-

Table 9.1 Examination strategy

Localizer pelvis, abdomen, lung
Rectum HASTE axial, coronal, sagittal for fine planning
Spasmolyticum (Buscopan i.v.)
Rectum T2-weighted, high resolution axial and sagittal
Liver T1-weighted, pre-contrast (3D VIBE sequence)
Liver T1-weighted, dynamic arterial and portal-venous
Lung T1-weighted, venous
Lung and liver T2-weighted
Full abdomen (HASTE)
Liver T1-weighted with fat saturation in liver-specific phase (Primovist®, 20 min post contrast)

Table 9.2 MRI rectum

Turbo spin-echo sequence	
TR	5420 ms
TE	84 ms
Flip angle	180°
Slice thickness	3.0 mm
Number of slices	23
Inter-slice separation (gap)	0
Field of view	160 mm
Acquisition time	5 min 32 s
Matrix	256 × 256
Local resolution	0.6 × 0.6 × 3.0 mm
Orientation	axial and sagittal

Table 9.3 Liver MRI

	Volume-interpolated breath-hold examination (3D VIBE)	2D gradient-echo sequence
TR	4.87 ms	152 ms
TE	2.33 ms	2.72 ms
Flip angle	10°	70°
Slice thickness	2.5 mm	7.0 mm
Number of slices	64	24
Inter-slice separation (gap)	/	10%
Field of view	350–400 mm	350–400 mm
Acquisition time	23 s	22 s
Matrix	125 × 256	145 × 256
Spatial resolution	at least 2,2 × 1,4 × 2,5 mm	at least 2,0 × 1,4 × 7,0 mm

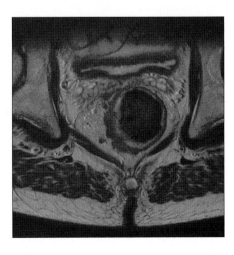

Figure 9.1 Whole-body MRI for staging a patient with histologically verified adenocarcinoma of the rectum. T2-weighted turbo spin-echo sequence in axial orientation. Wall thickening of the right-side and dorsal rectal wall with blurred boundary to perirectal fat tissue consistent with T3 stage. Presentation of two surrounding lymph nodes under 1 cm diameter. MR imaging stage T3N1.

Table 9.4 Lung MRI

	Volume-interpolated breath-hold examination (3D VIBE)	**T2 turbo spin-echo PACE**
TR	4.87 ms	1200 ms
TE	2.33 ms	70 ms
Flip angle	20°	150°
Slice thickness	2.5 mm	6.0 mm
Number of slices	64	42
Inter-slice separation (gap)	/	10%
Field of view	350–400 mm	350–400 mm
Acquisition time	23 s	approx. 2.37 min
Matrix	135 × 256	216 × 320
Local resolution	2.2 × 1,4 × 2.5 mm	1.3 × 1,2 × 6.0 mm
Orientation	axial	axial
Breathing	breath-hold	PACE respiratory triggering

quence (Fig. 9.2). As Primovist® has no influence on T2-weighted images and the liver-specific images are not acquired until after 20 min [13], the option is available of imaging the liver and lung with respiratory-triggered T2-weighted sequences. In addition, the entire abdomen and pelvis are imaged with a T2-weighted half-Fourier single-shot turbo spin-echo (HASTE) sequence to capture organ infiltration, pathologically enlarged lymph nodes, or metastases.

The acquisition of the liver-specific phase in axial and coronal orientation takes place after 20 min (Fig 9.3). Whole-body imaging with T1-weighting can be useful, especially for the documentation of the overall TNM stage (Fig. 9.4). The total examination period is around 45 min.

The highest accuracy for the detection and localization of liver metastases is offered in the liver-specific late phase; it is therefore also conceivable to forgo the liver dynamics in

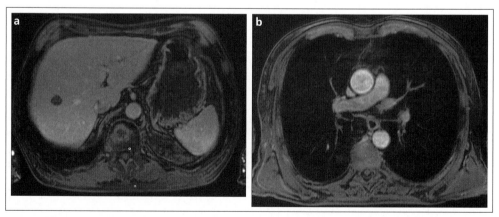

Figure 9.2a, b Liver in the portal-venous phase (3D VIBE sequence). Hypovascularized round metastasis in Segment 8 **(a)**. Lung in venous phase (approx. 30 s after contrast, 3D VIBE sequence). No evidence of lung nodules. Good contrasting of the vasculature after administration of liver-specific contrast agent Primovist® **(b).**

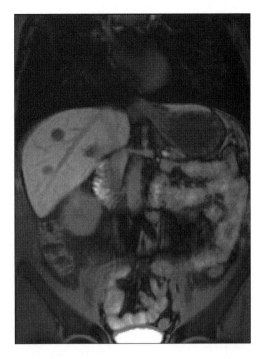

Figure 9.3 Coronal orientation through the liver in the liver-specific phase (20 min after administration of contrast agent). The high signal presentation of the hepatic parenchyma in the T1-weighted 2D GRE sequence through the specific uptake of Primovist® in the hepatocytes is clearly recognizable, while the 3 liver metastases appear hypointense. The high contrast between the hepatic parenchyma and metastases on the one hand, and the rapid washout of the contrast agent from the intravascular space on the other hand (identifiable from the hypointense portal vein), leads to an improvement not only in the detection of lesions, but also exact localization. The preoperative planning of metastasis resection is improved as a result.

the perfusion phase and instead to acquire the perfusion of the primary tumor after injection of Primovist®. However, the characterization of the discovered liver lesions (e.g. differential diagnosis metastasis/focal nodular hyperplasia) can become problematic, as the dynamic perfusion information of the lesion is missing [3].

The Primovist® protocol presented can also be applied in a similar form for staging other malignomas, e.g. colon carcinoma or stomach carcinoma.

9.3 Lymph node specific contrast agent

The new ultra-small superparamagnetic contrast agent Sinerem® (Guerbet, Paris/France) is still undergoing clinical trials. It is phagocytized by the reticuloendothelial system (RES), as are larger iron oxides. After intravenous application, the ultrasmall iron oxide particles (USPIOs) pass through the first lymphatic barriers (liver and spleen) due to their small diameter and their neutral electrical charge, and arrive in the lymph nodes, where they are phagocytized by the local macrophages.

The local concentration of iron oxide leads to a significant rise in the local T2 and T2* relaxivity [14–15].

Non-pathological lymph nodes therefore show a significant reduction in the T2 and T2* signal starting 1 hour after administration of the contrast agent. Pathological lymph nodes, for which the regular lymphatic tissue is displaced by the metastatic tissue, show no significant signal change due to the absence of macrophage activity. Promising results have been reported in the staging of solid tumors of the prostate and the larynx [16–20].

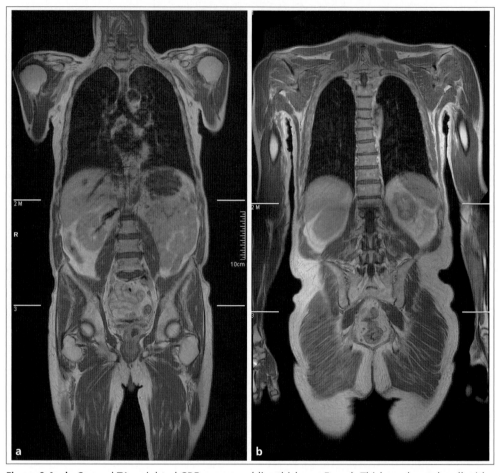

Figure 9.4a, b Coronal T1-weighted GRE sequence (slice thickness 5 mm). Thickened rectal wall with blurred boundary to the perirectal fat tissue, perirectal lymph nodes **(b)**, liver metastasis in Segment 8 **(a)**, no evidence of bone metastases. To summarize: rectal carcinoma stage T3N1 M1hep.

9.4 Whole-body MRI with lymph node specific contrast agent

Whole-body MRI opens up new perspectives, especially for lymph node staging (N status) of malignant tumors. Until now MRI has been primarily limited to the evaluation of regional lymph nodes. The identification of distant lymph node metastases is only possible with great effort, i.e. repositioning the patient and/or the exchange of coils. Also, the information on the infiltration of lymph nodes is not very specific, as the criteria consist of morphological parameters, such as size, ratio between longitudinal and transverse diameters, or homogeneity of the signal. Sensitivities of between 25 and 70% are stated in the literature for the identification of lymph node metastases. Especially lymph nodes with a diameter under 10 mm cannot be reliably assessed [17].

Whole-body MRI using USPIOs could succeed in overcoming both limitations. The diagnostic accuracy in the detection of metastasis-infiltrated lymph nodes increases, as functional information is available with the analysis of the USPIO image and the enhancement pattern alongside the morphological parameters. Whole-body technology allows the presentation of all lymph node stations within a reasonable period of time.

Initial experience is available in staging Hodgkin and non-Hodgkin lymph nodes. Patient management and the prognosis of both diseases are significantly affected by the extent of the disease, as well as by the clinical findings and the laboratory values. The staging of Hodgkin lymphomas takes place according to the Ann-Arbor criteria from 1971 and their modification by Cotswold from 1989 for non-Hodgkin lymphomas. Until now, this has primarily been determined on the basis of combined throat, thorax, abdomen, and pelvis CT examinations.

The whole-body MR imaging examination strategy with TIM technology (Siemens Magnetom Avanto, Siemens Medical Systems, Erlangen, Germany) includes coronal T1, T2 and T2* weighted sequences (Table 9.5). Matrix coils (24-channel spine coil, 12-channel head coil, 6-channel neck coil, two-three 6-channel body coils depending on the size of the patient, and 18-channel peripheral coil) are used. All sequences are performed consecutively at each level; 5–6 stations of each sequence are measured with a field of view (FOV) of 35–40 cm and an overlap of 20% and are then automatically combined ("Composing", Fig. 9.5). In addition, axial sequences of the neurocranium (e.g. T2-weighted turbo spin-echo sequences, fluid suppressed T2-weighted FLAIR sequence, T1-weighted spin-echo sequence) and axial T1 and T2-weighted sequences of the thorax and abdomen can be performed in breath-hold or using respiratory triggering.

All sequences are performed without contrast agent. The USPIOs are administered under medical supervision as slow infusions. The dose used is 2.6 mg iron/kg body weight. A time window of 24–36 h after application of the USPIOs is recommended as the ideal time for post-contrast imaging. Here the T2 and T2*-weighted sequences are performed using identical parameters as in the examination prior to administration of contrast agent, so that the uptake in lymph nodes and other tissue through RES activity can be evaluated both visually as well as quantitatively (Fig. 9.6). Additionally, the T1-weighted sequences should be repeated, because the USPIOs produce a high intravascular contrast effect even after 24–36 h, so that vessels can be imaged with a rich signal and are easy to distinguish from other structures, such as lymph nodes (Fig. 9.7). This intravascular contrast effect is caused by the particles still circulating in the blood. The USPIOs, as very small iron oxides, have a strong influence on the T1 relaxivity [21].

Table 9.5 Whole-body MRI examination for lymphoma staging

• T2-weighted fast spin-echo sequence (TR: 4000–4500 ms, TE: 80–100 ms, flip angle: 90°, coronal orientation, slice thickness 5 mm, slice separation 0.1 mm, 512×410 matrix, field of view: 5× (350–400 mm).
• T2*-weighted gradient-echo sequence (TR: 800–1500 ms, TE: 25 ms, flip angle: 30°, coronal orientation, slice thickness 5 mm, slice separation 0.1 mm, 256×160 matrix, field of view: 5× (350–400 mm).
• T1-weighted fast spin-echo sequence (TR: 400–600 ms, TE: 5–10 ms, flip angle: 90°, coronal orientation, slice thickness 5 mm, slice separation 0.1 mm, 512×410 matrix, field of view: 5× (350–400 mm).

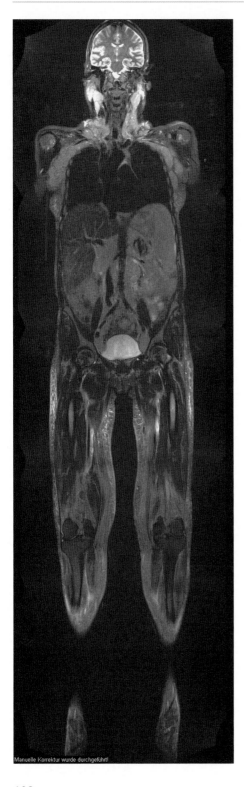

Manuelle Korrektur wurde durchgeführt!

Figure 9.5 Unenhanced fat suppressed T2-STIR sequence. Extended CLL (chronic lymphocytic leukemia) in a 53-year-old patient with extensive cervical, thoracic, abdominal, and pelvic lymph node conglomerates and splenomegaly.

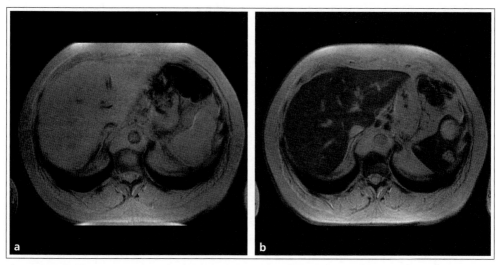

Figure 9.6a, b T2*-weighted gradient-echo sequence in axial orientation before **(a)** and after administration of Sinerem® **(b)**. Extended, confluent abdominal lymph node conglomerates which completely surround the abdominal aorta ("bulking disease"). Absorption in the liver and spleen is apparent 24 h after administration of the contrast agent. Several focal lymphoma lesions are visible in the spleen, which are not distinguishable in the unenhanced sequence. There is no change in the signal pattern for the bulking disease; only lymphoma tissue is present here. In the region of the lesser stomach curvature, several solitary lymph nodes, which on account of their size cannot be reliably classified as pathological, are shown with a significant and homogeneous signal change. These lymph nodes therefore display proper RES activity and are not infiltrated by lymphoma.

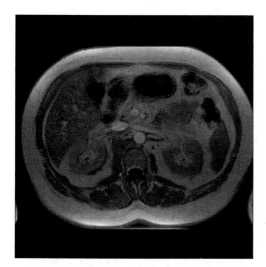

Figure 9.7 The same patient as in Fig. 9.6. T1-weighted turbo spin-echo sequence in axial orientation 24 h after administration of Sinerem®. Apparent is the intense intravascular contrast effect with identical signal intensity in the abdominal aorta, inferior vena cava, right renal vein, and the intrahepatic vessels. In this distribution phase, one speaks of a blood pool contrast effect.

Besides the previously published indications for use of Sinerem® (N staging with prostate carcinoma and ENT-related malignomas), the use of the contrast agent is also conceivable for staging numerous other tumor entities, e.g. gynecological malignomas (cervix carcinoma, endometrium carcinoma, ovarian carcinoma).

Bibliography

1. Hamm B, Staks T, Mühler A, Bollow M, Taupitz M, Frenzel T, Wolf K, Weinmann HJ, Lange L. Phase I clinical evaluation of Gd-EOB-DTPA as a hepatobiliary MR contrast agent: safety, pharmakokinetics, and MR imaging. Radiology 1995; 195: 785–92.
2. Huppertz A, Balzer T, Blakeborough A, Breuer J, Giovagnoni A, Heinz-Peer G, Laniado M et al. Improved detection of focal liver lesions at MR imaging: A multicenter comparison of gadoxetic acid-enhanced MR images with intraoperative findings. Radiology 2004; 230: 266–75.
3. Huppertz A, Haraida S, Kraus A, Zech CJ, Scheidler J, Breuer J, Helmberger TK, Reiser MF. Enhancement of focal liver lesions at gadoxetic acid-enhanced MR imaging: Correlation with histopathologic findings and spiral CT – initial observations. Radiology 2005; 234: 468–78.
4. Petersein J, Spinazzi A, Giovagnoni A, Soyer P et al. Focal liver lesions: evaluation of the efficacy of gadobenate dimeglumine in MR imaging – a multicenter phase III clinical study. Radiology 2000; 215: 727–36.
5. http://www.dkfz-heidelberg.de/tzhdma/tr28.htm
6. Laghi A, Ferri M, Catalano C, Baeli I, Iannaccone R, Iafrate F, Ziparo V, Passariello R. Local staging of rectal cancer with MRI using a phased array body coil. Abdom Imaging 2002 Jul–Aug; 27(4): 425–31.
7. Brown G, Daniels IR. Preoperative staging of rectal cancer: the MERCURY research project. Recent Results Cancer Res 2005; 165: 58–74.
8. Strassburg J. Magnetic resonance imaging in rectal cancer: the MERCURY experience. Tech Coloproctol 2004 Nov; 8 Suppl 1: 16–8.
9. Brown G, Richards CJ, Newcombe RG, Dallimore NS, Radcliffe AG, Carey DP, Bourne MW, Williams GT. Rectal carcinoma: thin-section MR imaging for staging in 28 patients. Radiology 1999 Apr; 211(1): 215–22.
10. Bissett IP, Fernando CC, Hough DM, Cowan BR, Chau KY, Young AA, Parry BR, Hill GL. Identification of the fascia propria by magnetic resonance imaging and its relevance to preoperative assessment of rectal cancer. Dis Colon Rectum 2001 Feb; 44(2): 259–65.
11. Vliegen RF, Beets GL, von Meyenfeldt MF, Kessels AG, Lemaire EE, van Engelshoven JM, Beets-Tan RG. Rectal cancer: MR imaging in local staging – is gadolinium-based contrast material helpful? Radiology 2005 Jan; 234(1): 179–88.
12. Schafer JF, Vollmar J, Schick F, Seemann MD, Kamm P, Erdtmann B, Claussen CD. Detection of pulmonary nodules with breath-hold magnetic resonance imaging in comparison with computed tomography. Rofo 2005 ; 177: 41–9.
13. Reimer P, Rummeny EJ, Daldrup HE, Hesse T, Balzer T, Tombach B, Peters PE. Enhancement characteristics of liver metastases, hepatocellular carcinomas, and hemangiomas with Gd-EOB-DTPA: preliminary results with dynamic MR imaging. Eur Radiol 1997; 7: 275–80.
14. Mack MG, Balzer JO, Straub R, Eichler K, Vogl TJ. Superparamagnetic iron oxide-enhanced MR imaging of head and neck lymph nodes. Radiology 2002; 222: 239–44.
15. Bellin MF, Lebleu L, Meric JB. Evaluation of retroperitoneal and pelvic lymph node metastases with MRI and MR lymphangiography. Abdom Imaging 2003; 28: 155–63.
16. Beyersdorff D, Taupitz M, Giessing M, et al. [The staging of bladder tumors in MRT: the value of the intravesical application of an iron oxide-containing contrast agent in combination with high-resolution T2-weighted imaging]. Rofo 2000; 172: 504–8.

17. Jager GJ, Barentsz JO, Oosterhof GO, Witjes JA, Ruijs SJ. Pelvic adenopathy in prostatic and urinary bladder carcinoma: MR imaging with a three-dimensional TI-weighted magnetizationprepared rapid gradient-echo sequence. AJR Am J Roentgenol 1996; 167: 1503–7.

18. Koh DM, Brown G, Temple L, et al. Rectal cancer: mesorectal lymph nodes at MR imaging with USPIO versus histopathologic findings – initial observations. Radiology 2004; 231: 91–9.

19. Deserno WM, Harisinghani MG, Taupitz M, et al. Urinary bladder cancer: preoperative nodal staging with ferumoxtran-10-enhanced MR imaging. Radiology 2004; 233: 449–56.

20. Harisinghani MG, Barentsz J, Hahn PF, et al. Noninvasive detection of clinically occult lymphnode metastases in prostate cancer. N Engl J Med 2003; 348: 2491–9.

21. Bremer C, Allkemper T, Baemig J, Reimer P. RES-specific imaging of the liver and spleen with iron oxide particles designed for blood-pool MR-angiography. J Magn Reson Imaging 1999; 10: 461–7.

10 Whole-body fat measurement

Florian M. Vogt

10.1 Introduction

Obesity, as an expression of a raised body fat proportion, represents an increasing health problem in the western world with growing prevalence [1]. Studies recently conducted in the US have revealed that more than half of all adults are overweight. Although the body fat plays an important role in the metabolic process as a source of aerobic energy during low intensity, prolonged activity, a raised proportion of body fat often has negative health implications [2]. The risks correlated with obesity have formed the basis of many studies. A consequence of increased fat in the aging population is a change in total weight and the ratio of active body substances (muscular system and bone structure) compared to body fat. It could be shown that even persons with an ideal weight for their age still increase their fat and reduce their muscle with age. This development may be accompanied by an impairment of muscular function and physical constitution. Furthermore, cardiovascular, endocrinological, gastroenterological, and neoplastic disease have been shown to correlate with obesity and represent a frequent cause of death [3–5]. Determination of the body fat provides information on the active body substance (muscular system and bone structure). In an effort to optimize measurement of the body fat, various methods have been developed, such as calipermetry, densitometry, infrared measurement, impedance measurement, and DEXA (dual-energy X-ray absorptiometry). All these methods allow improved evaluation of the body composition than a simple body composition index, e.g. the body mass index (BMI) or the BROCA index, which both simply reflect the relationship between body height and body mass with differentiated dimensionality of body height [6]. All these methods provide more or less sufficiently reliable information on total body fat; however, a detailed differentiation and quantification of subcutaneous and visceral storage fat is not possible. Recent studies indicate that mainly visceral storage fat, which differs morphologically and metabolically from subcutaneous fatty tissue, appears to play an important role in the pathogenesis of insulin regulation, dyslipidemias, hypertension, coronary heart disease (CHD), as well as ovarian and colon carcinoma [7–16]. However, it is not only the ratio of visceral to subcutaneous fat, but also the quantification of regional fat reserves in the different regions of the body that is of clinical and scientific interest. Changes in and control of diet, on the one hand, and training programs, on the other, are of increasing importance in the evaluation of total body fat and its distribution [17].

Modern cross-sectional imaging, such as computed tomography (CT) and magnetic resonance imaging (MRI), allow differentiation and determination of visceral and subcutaneous fat in all regions of the body [18–19]. The accuracy of both methods has been evaluated in vivo with different models and shows excellent correlations [20–24]. Whereas CT is only permitted for a limited number of individual measurements on account of the accompanying radiation exposure, MRI not only allows whole-body acquisition, but also the option of repeated progress monitoring [17, 25–28]. The goal of this article is to provide an overview of the options for determining body fat. Taking current technical advancements into consideration, various MRI techniques to determine the fat reserve and its distribution are discussed, and an efficient examination protocol for whole-body fat measurement is proposed.

10.2 Comparison of methods for determining whole-body fat content

10.2.1 Anthropometric methods

The starting point is the division of the whole body into so-called compartments. According to the two-compartment model, body mass can be divided into fat mass and fat-free mass. This dichotomic division is indeed strongly simplified, but has proven its worth as the basis for fat measurement.

The simplest method is calipermetry. The portions of the body fat are determined at various places on the basis of measurement of the skin fold thickness with orientation from morphological features. The doubled skin folds are measured with a caliper by lifting the skin with forefinger and thumb [29]. Prescribed measurement rules make an examination easy to perform, but its reliability depends on the experience of the practitioner. The method is subject to several possible sources of error. The caliper is to be placed with a contact pressure of 10 g/mm². The thickness of the skin fold must be read off within 4 s to avoid compression of the fat tissue. The measurement error is 3–11% and is furthermore influenced by age and gender [30]. However, this method is inexpensive, widely available, and its low level of technical complexity and easy performance justify its use for non-scientific applications.

10.2.2 Classical laboratory methods

10.2.2.1 Densitometry

Densitometry involves determining body density with underwater weighing. This is given by the formula: Body density (g/cm³) = body mass (g)/body volume (cm³). The fat and non-fat masses are determined from the ratio of body mass to body volume. A densitometric examination is very time-consuming. For example, the determination of the body volume is dependent on the residual volume of the lung, so that the residual air must be determined prior to underwater weighing to obtain the most accurate density value possible. This technique is chosen for selected examinations in a laboratory with a water tank. A good correlation has been described between densitometry and DEXA, CT, and MRI in the measurement of total body fat [31, 32].

10.2.2.2 Hydrometry

Body water determination is often chosen in the evaluation of body composition and is based on the dilution principle of fluids (blood). Analyses of this type often use deuterium [33]. It is based on the assumption that body water makes up a constant proportion of

73.2% of the fat-free body mass. The correlation between body mass and total body water is very high at r = 0.96–0.99. This method is only possible at technically well-equipped laboratories with qualified personnel. The measurement accuracy is high.

10.2.2.3 Bioelectric impedance analysis (BIA)

BIA is an electrical resistance measurement with which the electrical conductance of the organism is determined [34]. The devices used generate a homogeneous electrical field with constant current and high frequency in the person undergoing measurement. The total body fluid can be concluded from the electrical resistance (impedance) that the body presents. Lean muscle tissue has a higher electrical conductivity than fat tissue on account of the higher fluid and electrolyte content, so that the fat and lean mass in the organism can be derived with the use of a low current passed through the body and the resistance that arises. Although some studies show good agreement in the quantification of fat mass between BIA and other more direct methods, insufficient knowledge of the scientific and methodological background of fat determination with BIA must be emphasized [35]. The measurement conditions must be kept constant to obtain reliable results. The influential internal and external factors in the impedance method appear wide-ranging. These include the fluid balance of the organism, on which the impedance measurement is based, which cannot be easily ascertained. Alcohol consumption, a full stomach, or a full bladder can lead to falsified results, as can sweating or temperature changes in the hands and feet.

10.2.2.4 Infrared measurement

Infrared measurement is based on the different absorption of infrared radiation. Whereas the absorption maximum for fat is at a wavelength of 930 nm, water absorbs infrared radiation up to 970 nm. A well-known device is the Futrex, which is placed on the skin of the dominant upper arm (biceps) [36]. Near-infrared illumination takes place during the measurement, with which the optical density of the tissue is determined. This is taken to analyze the fat proportion of the organism by means of an estimation function while taking age, fitness, gender, body weight, as well as bone structure into consideration. The measurement accuracy still requires detailed scientific investigation. The measurement accuracy is apparently around 2%.

10.2.2.5 Dual energy X-ray absorptiometry (DEXA)

The use of the DEXA method to evaluate total body fat content has become widely established due to its easy applicability, rapid examination procedure, and low costs. The principle of the method is based on the three-component model, which differentiates between fat tissue, lean tissue, and bone [37–39]. These attenuate the applied low dosage X-rays (effective dose < 5 µSv for whole-body examination) to varying degrees. Advances in hardware and software have brought about a multitude of studies investigating the differences between the respective devices [40, 41]. The DEXA method is often taken as the standard of reference for the evaluation of new methods of body fat determination [42]. Nevertheless, this method also presents several sources of error. Variable hydration of the lean mass leads to incorrect calculation of the proportion of fat. Moreover, it must be considered that this method measures all fat components, i.e. also essential fat occurring in the bone marrow,

CNS, heart, lungs, liver, spleen, kidneys, as well as intramuscular fat, and can therefore lead to false-positive results. As with all the techniques presented so far, the DEXA method is also not in a position to differentiate between visceral and subcutaneous fat tissue.

10.3 Methods for determining regional fat reserves and total whole-body fat content

10.3.1 Computed tomography

Computed tomography, which excels by virtue of its detailed depiction of visceral and subcutaneous fat, appears unsuitable for presenting the total body fat due to its radiation exposure. Kvist et al. determined an effective dose of 2–4 mSv for the acquisition of 22 slices [27]. Even given a reduction in the radiation dose through the application of low-dose CT protocols, the number of measurements on one person is limited and makes this method appear unsuitable for follow-up and long-term examinations. Although studies reveal that the quantity of visceral fat which was determined from CT in a single acquired slice correlates well with the results obtained from several acquired slices, the use of single slice methods can cause measurement error due to intestinal sections and partial volume effects [18, 43]. The amount of visceral and/or subcutaneous fat also varies very strongly between individuals, which increases the difficulty in estimating the total visceral and subcutaneous fat using the single slice technique [28]. Assessment of the reduction or redistribution of fat reserves to different regions of the body as a result of dietary or exercise programs is not possible at all due to the concomitant radiation exposure.

10.3.2 Magnetic resonance imaging

The advantages of MRI lie in the absence of radiation exposure, as well as in the high resolution of anatomical detail and the good depictability and differentiation of both bone and soft tissue structures. Fat tissue has the highest MRI signal intensity of all tissues in the body. The protons bound in fat molecules have a 3.5 ppm lower resonance frequency than water-bound protons, and the reduced longitudinal relaxation time T1 of the lipid components in T1-weighted imaging becomes clearly significant and allows easy differentiation from the other soft tissue. The development of measurement sequences in recent years has led to a wide range of techniques with T1-weighted contrast. The clinical MRI systems started with spin-echo sequences (single, double, inversion recovery), which were widely used in fat measurement. Many studies have demonstrated both in vivo as well as in vitro the accuracy of MRI in determining fat mass as compared with CT, DEXA, and underwater measurement [32, 39, 44–46]. Classical spin-echo sequences, however, require several minutes for acquisition of one region of the body. As a consequence of this technical limitation, the use of MRI for whole-body diagnostics was only possible to a limited extent, because, to complete a whole-body examination, several sequences have to be combined such that the examination times > 30 min are attained. Taking the compromise between costs (including acquisition and evaluation time) and the accuracy of the method into consideration, only a single slice technique with subsequent extrapolation or multi-slice techniques on selected regions of the body were applied in analogy to CT [18, 44, 47]. These methods, however, exclude the aforementioned option of evaluating the relationship between different body fat reserves under certain dietary and exercise programs, as well as growth conditions. Furthermore, they show the same potential measurement errors caused by interpolation as single-slice CT techniques. With the exception of the absence of radiation exposure, no further advantages are offered.

Newly developed fast spin-echo sequences and gradient-echo sequences have overcome this problem [17, 48]. While fast spin-echo sequences use a multiple signal read-out following single excitation, gradient-echo sequences use a partial deflection of the spin from the magnetic field axis to achieve significantly faster repeated excitation and readout. These techniques allow acquisition of a region of the body with the breath holding technique and today are the imaging methods of choice for whole-body fat measurements.

Fast spin-echo sequences and gradient-echo sequences also show considerably fewer artifacts as compared with classical spin-echo sequences.

As a result of the inherently high signal from fat tissue, fat measurement is also possible using MRI scanner generations with low-power gradient systems. The integrated body coil is entirely adequate for signal reception; special surface coils are not required.

10.3.3 Whole-body MR fat measurement

The concept of whole-body fat measurement is based on the capture of several sequential 2D data sets in direct chronological order as far as possible. The entire body from the hands to the ankles is acquired in this case (Fig. 10.1). To ensure both fast, time-effective acquisition of these data sets, as well as optimal image quality, a few aspects have to be considered:

Due to the limited field of view of the scanner, the arms of the person examined should be placed over the head. This does increase the volume to be covered implying an increase in the total acquisition time; however, aliasing artifacts from the arms and inhomogeneities on the margins of the image are reduced. This technique has proven itself, especially for corpulent patients whose arms could not be captured when placed on the trunk. The subsequent evaluation using semi-automated software is far easier, and the accuracy of the measurement method increases. Furthermore, data acquisition of the respective body region to be examined should take place at the isocenter of the magnet, as significant distortions can arise with increasing distance from the center [48]. If these aspects are taken into account, overlapping acquisition of the data sets is not necessary. However, as a rule, the range of movement of the scanner table is not sufficiently long to meet the demands of whole-body imaging. Two techniques are in principle applicable to still allow complete capture of the

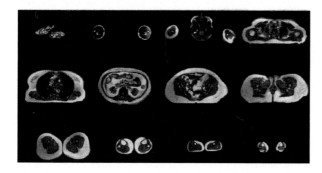

Figure 10.1 Single slices from a whole-body measurement of a volunteer.

body volume. In the first technique, the person examined has to be repositioned on the scanning table such that the upper half of the body volume (arms first into the scanner) and subsequently the lower half of the body (feet first into the scanner) are captured [17]. But this technique is more time-consuming and is subject to measurement inaccuracy arising from repositioning and the resulting overlapping or missing data acquisition. In the second method, the person is placed on a roller-mounted table platform (Body*SURF*, MR-Innovation GmbH, Essen, Germany, see Chap. 1), mounted on the original patient table [49]. The platform is moved continuously in this process and thereby allows complete capture of the complete body volume without the necessity of repositioning.

10.3.4 MRI protocol

The planning and performance of whole-body fat measurement by means of a turbo spin-echo or gradient-echo sequence is not complicated. Special attention must only be paid to ensuring the seamless capture of the individual regions.

As the volumes captured in the field of view show significantly varying characteristics (e.g. data set from the arms vs. upper abdomen), shimming and tuning should be carried out prior to capturing the respective data sets to obtain homogeneous signal intensity in the respective volume.

10.3.5 MRI sequences

The longitudinal relaxation time of protons bound to free water in a field strength of 1.5 T is 1100 ms, whereas the T1 time of protons bound in fat tissue is roughly 270 ms. The repetition time (TR) and echo time (TE) should be selected in spin-echo and gradient-echo sequences such that a maximum separation of fat and soft tissue is achieved. As short an echo time as possible is desirable due to the short T2 relaxation time of fat tissue. The repetition time, matched to the flip angle, should also be selected to be short. The fat tissue with its bound protons is then available for repeated excitation, whereas substances in which the effect of the initial excitation remains for a long period do not yet contribute to the imaging signal again. As gradient-echo sequences, unlike spin-echo sequences, do not use a 180° pulse, short echo times and also correspondingly short repetition times are possible. In gradient-echo sequences, a lower flip angle is also to be set to match the shorter TR to avoid saturation of the fat tissue. Due to the use of a 180° pulse and inherently longer echo times, spin-echo sequences show a more homogeneous signal since field inhomogeneities are partially compensated. For MRI scanners with a lower field strength, the T1 relaxation times are shorter, so that the echo and repetition times, as well as the flip angle, have to be adapted. In principle, the field of view (FOV) can be adapted to the respective body region to be examined. The necessary planning for this takes time, though. As the capture of fat tissue is not subject to a time limiting factor, as in the case of whole-body MR angiography, it is sufficient to select the field of view and the parameters for all regions such that the largest volumes of the body (chest and abdomen) are fully captured and can be acquired within a single breath-holding phase.

The most accurate MRI methods for determining whole-body fat would be, without doubt, those with which the entire body volume is captured without gaps. This however would lead to a significant increase in the overall acquisition time and would prevent the coverage of large volumes in a single breath-holding phase. The necessity would therefore arise of capturing many sequences, each covering a small volume. Furthermore, seamless acquisition would lead to a flood of data, which would consequently prolong the evaluation phase considerably. The partial omission of slices from a contiguous data set reduces the acquisition and evaluation time, but leads to a successive reduction in the degree of accuracy as the number of omitted slices is increased. A compromise must therefore be found between the accuracy of a technique and the acquisition/evaluation time.

Using a fast spin-echo sequence with a TR/TE of 490/12 ms, a flip angle of 90°, a slice thickness of 10 mm, a slice separation of 10 mm, a FOV of 450–500 mm and a matrix of 178×256, capture of 5 slices per sequence is possible in 12 s. The total acquisition time is 20–25 min [17].

Faster data capture is possible using the roller-mounted table platform. Using a 2D Flash sequence with a TR/TE of 101/4.7 ms, a flip angle of 70°, a slice thickness of 10 mm, a slice separation of 10 mm, a FOV of 500×500 mm and a matrix of 205×256, a data set consisting of 10 slices per sequence can be captured in 20 s. The examination table is moved within a 3 s long pause between the individual stations. A maximum total acquisition time of 227 s results for 8–10 body stations. The whole-body MR fat measurement including positioning of the subject can be performed in approx. 10–15 min [50]. The examination protocol has shown itself to be robust.

10.3.6 Data analysis

After transmission of the acquired data sets to a separate PC, evaluation takes place using semi-automated software which uses a contour-tracking algorithm (Fig. 10.2). After the initial creation of a grey-level histogram, two threshold values are determined, whereby the first serves to differentiate the inherent background noise in the image from pixels containing information on the body volume. The second threshold value distinguishes fat from fat-free tissue (Fig. 10.3). Each slice is then visually checked and can, if necessary, be corrected by interactively changing the second threshold value. This option needs be integrated into the software to be able to exclude pixels from the evaluation which can show the same signal patterns as fat tissue, e.g. within the hepatic parenchyma or the content of the intestines.

The volume of tissue (cm³) is then calculated by multiplying the corresponding area (image pixels) with the slice thickness and the number of slices. If the separation between two acquired slices within a data set corresponds to the slice thickness, the total volume of a data set can be calculated by simple duplication. The following volumes can be evaluated: whole-body volume, whole-body fat tissue, volumes of subcutaneous and visceral fat tissue (Figs. 10.4 and 10.5).

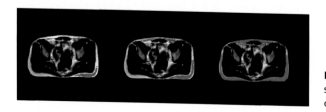

Figure 10.2 Functionality of the semi-automated software using a contour-tracking algorithm..

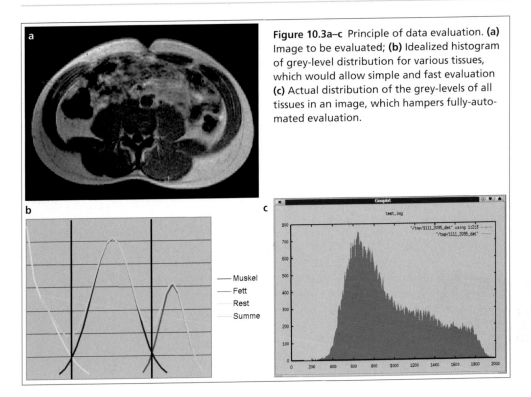

Figure 10.3a–c Principle of data evaluation. **(a)** Image to be evaluated; **(b)** Idealized histogram of grey-level distribution for various tissues, which would allow simple and fast evaluation **(c)** Actual distribution of the grey-levels of all tissues in an image, which hampers fully-automated evaluation.

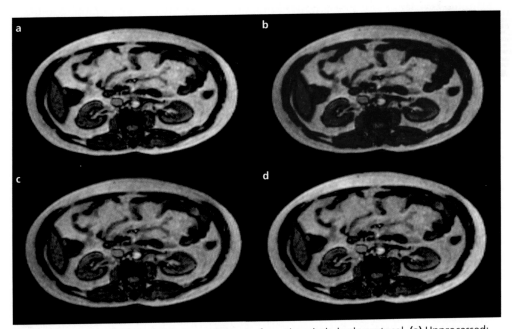

Figure 10.4a–d Single slice of the upper abdomen from the whole-body protocol. **(a)** Unprocessed; **(b)** Determination of the total volume; **(c)** Quantification of subcutaneous and visceral fat tissue; **(d)** Quantification of just the visceral fat tissue.

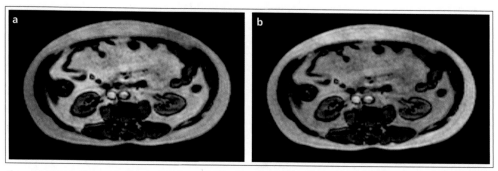

Figure 10.5a, b Separate determination of **(a)** subcutaneous and **(b)** visceral fat tissue.

This method allows direct measurement of the volume of fat tissue, but does not specify the absolute mass of triglycerides contained in the fat tissue. In many studies, however, the fat mass is taken for comparison with other methods. Fat tissue consists of 80% triglycerides, 2% proteins, and 18% water and minerals and has an average density of 0.9255 kg/l [51]. The amount of fat can therefore be determined from the following equation:

Fat volume $\times 0.9255 \times 80\%$.

10.3.7 Problems of MRI whole-body fat measurement

Due to longer imaging times, spin-echo sequences are generally more susceptible to breathing, peristaltic, and pulse-induced motion artifacts. In addition to motion-induced blurring from the movement of organs during the image capture time, potential signal changes arise with the ingestion of saturated or unsaturated fluids or intestinal motility, which can be misinterpreted as fat tissue. Only smaller volumes can therefore be covered in the breath-holding technique, as compared with gradient-echo sequences, to reduce these artifacts. The data sets nevertheless show a more homogeneous signal pattern. Donelly et al. succeeded in demonstrating that turbo spin-echo sequences allow more accurate determination of the total amount of subcutaneous and visceral fat tissue than gradient-echo sequences [52].

However, determination of the ratio of visceral to subcutaneous fat tissue is equally successful with both methods. Although accurate determination of subcutaneous or visceral fat is of special importance for some studies, the ratio of the two types of reserve fat is taken for most determinations to ascertain the influence of risk factors. The former should be used for the precise evaluation of certain regions of the body, whereas in most cases the latter offers the more time-effective and therefore also the more cost-effective alternative.

A further problem which can influence the accuracy of the methods is presented by the gaps between the individual slices within a data set. These indeed enable fast capture of data sets using the breath-holding technique and therefore increase the effectiveness of the methods, while reducing the evaluation time by reducing the quantity of acquired data. But the inaccuracy of the measurement rises sharply with an increase in the gaps. Nevertheless, Thomas et al. managed to show that the deviation from a continuously acquired data set for capturing data sets with 10 mm thick slices and 10 mm gaps is very low in the evaluation of fat tissue [28].

The use of semi-automated software in the data analysis of a whole-body fat examination succeeded in significantly reducing the evaluation time from initially 4–5 hours to 15–30 min; nonetheless, considering the quantity of data and the personnel required, fully-automated evaluation would be preferable. Furthermore, measurement errors can also arise due to the individual selection of the threshold values for subcutaneous and visceral fat.

10.4 Current developments

In the last two years, a 1.5 Tesla MRI system (Avanto, Siemens Medical Systems, Erlangen, Germany) equipped with a whole-body coil system (76 coil elements) and 32 radiofrequency channels has been available with which a whole-body examination can be performed in a short time at high spatial resolution with a 205 cm field of view. Whereas a high spatial resolution is of major importance for many examination protocols and clinical investigations, this is of minor importance in whole-body fat measurement due to the inherently high signal for fat tissue. However, the large FOV allows in most cases complete capture of the fat tissue without repositioning or the necessity of additional technical equipment. This point aside, though, scanners of the previous and earlier generations offer sufficiently high accuracy in the evaluation of whole-body fat tissue.

10.5 Summary

Obesity represents a major health problem in the western countries with increasing prevalence. Not only the total quantity of body fat plays a crucial role in the pathogenesis of various diseases, but also its regional distribution. Magnetic resonance imaging allows a fast, non-invasive, whole-body examination with accurate determination of the ratio between subcutaneous and visceral fat reserves. The protocols and programs deployed facilitate quantification within 30–45 min. The techniques described here should be of assistance in determining the influence of genetic and environmental factors on the various body fat compartments.

Bibliography

1. Mokdad AH, Bowman BA, Ford ES, Vinicor F, Marks JS, Koplan JP. The continuing epidemics of obesity and diabetes in the United States. Jama 2001; 286: 1195–1200.
2. Baumgartner RN. Body composition in healthy aging. Ann N Y Acad Sci 2000; 904: 437–48.
3. Gautier JF, Mourier A, de Kerviler E, et al. Evaluation of abdominal fat distribution in noninsulin-dependent diabetes mellitus: relationship to insulin resistance. J Clin Endocrinol Metab 1998; 83: 1306–11.
4. Bjorntorp P. "Portal" adipose tissue as a generator of risk factors for cardiovascular disease and diabetes. Arteriosclerosis 1990; 10: 493–6.
5. Lemieux S, Despres JP, Moorjani S, et al. Are gender differences in cardiovascular disease risk factors explained by the level of visceral adipose tissue? Diabetologia 1994; 37: 757–64.
6. Chan DC, Watts GF, Barrett PH, Burke V. Waist circumference, waist-to-hip ratio and body mass index as predictors of adipose tissue compartments in men. Qjm 2003; 96: 441–7.

7. Despres JP, Nadeau A, Tremblay A, et al. Role of deep abdominal fat in the association between regional adipose tissue distribution and glucose tolerance in obese women. Diabetes 1989; 38: 304–9.

8. Kissebah AH, Peiris AN. Biology of regional body fat distribution: relationship to non-insulin-dependent diabetes mellitus. Diabetes Metab Rev 1989; 5: 83–109.

9. Kissebah AH, Vydelingum N, Murray R, et al. Relation of body fat distribution to metabolic complications of obesity. J Clin Endocrinol Metab 1982; 54: 254–60.

10. Krotkiewski M, Bjorntorp P, Sjostrom L, Smith U. Impact of obesity on metabolism in men and women. Importance of regional adipose tissue distribution. J Clin Invest 1983; 72: 1150–62.

11. Goodpaster BH, Krishnaswami S, Resnick H, et al. Association between regional adipose tissue distribution and both type 2 diabetes and impaired glucose tolerance in elderly men and women. Diabetes Care 2003; 26: 372–9.

12. Goodpaster BH, Krishnaswami S, Harris TB, et al. Obesity, regional body fat distribution, and the metabolic syndrome in older men and women. Arch Intern Med 2005; 165: 777–83.

13. Goran MI, Gower BA. Relation between visceral fat and disease risk in children and adolescents. Am J Clin Nutr 1999; 70: 149–56.

14. Rebuffe-Scrive M, Enk L, Crona N, et al. Fat cell metabolism in different regions in women. Effect of menstrual cycle, pregnancy, and lactation. J Clin Invest 1985; 75: 1973–6.

15. Wajchenberg BL. Subcutaneous and visceral adipose tissue: their relation to the metabolic syndrome. Endocr Rev 2000; 21: 697–738.

16. Garfinkel L. Overweight and cancer. Ann Intern Med 1985; 103: 1034–36.

17. Machann J, Thamer C, Schnoedt B, et al. Standardized assessment of whole body adipose tissue topography by MRI. J Magn Reson Imaging 2005; 21: 455–62.

18. Seidell JC, Bakker CJ, van der Kooy K. Imaging techniques for measuring adipose-tissue distribution – a comparison between computed tomography and 1.5-T magnetic resonance. Am J Clin Nutr 1990; 51: 953–7.

19. van der Kooy K, Seidell JC. Techniques for the measurement of visceral fat: a practical guide. Int J Obes Relat Metab Disord 1993; 17: 187–96.

20. Rossner S, Bo WJ, Hiltbrandt E, et al. Adipose tissue determinations in cadavers – a comparison between cross-sectional planimetry and computed tomography. Int J Obes 1990; 14: 893–902.

21. Ross R, Leger L, Guardo R, De Guise J, Pike BG. Adipose tissue volume measured by magnetic resonance imaging and computerized tomography in rats. J Appl Physiol 1991; 70: 2164–72.

22. Abate N, Burns D, Peshock RM, Garg A, Grundy SM. Estimation of adipose tissue mass by magnetic resonance imaging: validation against dissection in human cadavers. J Lipid Res 1994; 35: 1490–6.

23. Mitsiopoulos N, Baumgartner RN, Heymsfield SB, Lyons W, Gallagher D, Ross R. Cadaver validation of skeletal muscle measurement by magnetic resonance imaging and computerized tomography. J Appl Physiol 1998; 85: 115–22.

24. Fowler PA, Fuller MF, Glasbey CA, Cameron GG, Foster MA. Validation of the in vivo measurement of adipose tissue by magnetic resonance imaging of lean and obese pigs. Am J Clin Nutr 1992; 56: 7–13.

25. Sjostrom L. A computer-tomography based multicompartment body composition technique and anthropometric predictions of lean body mass, total and subcutaneous adipose tissue. Int J Obes 1991; 15 Suppl 2: 19–30.

26. Sjostrom L, Kvist H, Cederblad A, Tylen U. Determination of total adipose tissue and body fat in women by computed tomography, 40K, and tritium. Am J Physiol 1986; 250: E736–45.

27. Kvist H, Sjostrom L, Tylen U. Adipose tissue volume determinations in women by computed tomography: technical considerations. Int J Obes 1986; 10: 53–67.

28. Thomas EL, Saeed N, Hajnal JV, et al. Magnetic resonance imaging of total body fat. J Appl Physiol 1998; 85: 1778–85.

29. Durnin JV, Womersley J. Body fat assessed from total body density and its estimation from skinfold thickness: measurements on 481 men and women aged from 16 to 72 years. Br J Nutr 1974; 32: 77–97.

30. Wang J, Thornton JC, Kolesnik S, Pierson RN, Jr. Anthropometry in body composition. An overview. Ann N Y Acad Sci 2000; 904: 317–26.

31. Lockner DW, Heyward VH, Baumgartner RN, Jenkins KA. Comparison of air-displacement plethysmography, hydrodensitometry, and dual X-ray absorptiometry for assessing body composition of children 10 to 18 years of age. Ann N Y Acad Sci 2000; 904: 72–8.

32. McNeill G, Fowler PA, Maughan RJ, et al. Body fat in lean and overweight women estimated by six methods. Br J Nutr 1991; 65: 95–103.

33. Schoeller DA, van Santen E, Peterson DW, Dietz W, Jaspan J, Klein PD. Total body water measurement in humans with 18O and 2H labeled water. Am J Clin Nutr 1980; 33: 2686–93.

34. Deurenberg P, Weststrate JA, van der Kooy K. Body composition changes assessed by bioelectrical impedance measurements. Am J Clin Nutr 1989; 49: 401–3.

35. Schoeller DA. Bioelectrical impedance analysis. What does it measure? Ann N Y Acad Sci 2000; 904: 159–62.

36. Brooke-Wavell K, Jones PR, Norgan NG, Hardman AE. Evaluation of near infra-red interactance for assessment of subcutaneous and total body fat. Eur J Clin Nutr 1995; 49: 57–65.

37. Mazess RB, Barden HS, Bisek JP, Hanson J. Dual-energy X-ray absorptiometry for total-body and regional bone-mineral and soft-tissue composition. Am J Clin Nutr 1990; 51: 1106–12.

38. Tothill P. Dual-energy X-ray absorptiometers (DXA). Bone 1996; 19: 415–7.

39. Tothill P, Han TS, Avenell A, McNeill G, Reid DM. Comparisons between fat measurements by dual-energy X-ray absorptiometry, underwater weighing and magnetic resonance imaging in healthy women. Eur J Clin Nutr 1996; 50: 747–52.

40. Nord RH, Homuth JR, Hanson JA, Mazess RB. Evaluation of a new DXA fan-beam instrument for measuring body composition. Ann N Y Acad Sci 2000; 904: 118–25.

41. Mazess RB, Barden HS. Evaluation of differences between fan-beam and pencil-beam densitometers. Calcif Tissue Int 2000; 67: 291–6.

42. Jensen MD, Kanaley JA, Reed JE, Sheedy PF. Measurement of abdominal and visceral fat with computed tomography and dual-energy X-ray absorptiometry. Am J Clin Nutr 1995; 61: 274–8.

43. Kvist H, Chowdhury B, Grangard U, Tylen U, Sjostrom L. Total and visceral adipose-tissue volumes derived from measurements with computed tomography in adult men and women: predictive equations. Am J Clin Nutr 1988; 48: 1351–61.

44. Fowler PA, Fuller MF, Glasbey CA, et al. Total and subcutaneous adipose tissue in women: the measurement of distribution and accurate prediction of quantity by using magnetic resonance imaging. Am J Clin Nutr 1991; 54: 18–25.

45. Fuller MF, Fowler PA, McNeill G, Foster MA. Body composition: the precision and accuracy of new methods and their suitability for longitudinal studies. Proc Nutr Soc 1990; 49: 423–36.

46. Ross R, Shaw KD, Martel Y, de Guise J, Avruch L. Adipose tissue distribution measured by magnetic resonance imaging in obese women. Am J Clin Nutr 1993; 57: 470–5.

47. Abate N, Garg A, Coleman R, Grundy SM, Peshock RM. Prediction of total subcutaneous abdominal, intraperitoneal, and retroperitoneal adipose tissue masses in men by a single axial magnetic resonance imaging slice. Am J Clin Nutr 1997; 65: 403–8.

48. Barnard ML, Schwieso JE, Thomas EL, et al. Development of a rapid and efficient magnetic resonance imaging technique for analysis of body fat distribution. NMR Biomed 1996; 9: 156–64.

49. Lauenstein TC, Goehde SC, Herborn CU, et al. Whole-body MR imaging: evaluation of patients for metastases. Radiology 2004; 233: 139–48.

50. Vogt FM, Hunold P, de Greiff A, Ladd ME, Debatin JF, Ruehm SG. Total body fat quantification by magnetic resonance imaging. In: ECR. Wien, Austria; 2003: 293.

51. Thomas LW. The chemical composition of adipose tissue of man and mice. Q J Exp Physiol Cogn Med Sci 1962; 47: 179–88.

52. Donnelly LF, O'Brien KJ, Dardzinski BJ, et al. Using a phantom to compare MR techniques for determining the ratio of intraabdominal to subcutaneous adipose tissue. AJR Am J Roentgenol 2003; 180: 993–8.

11 Oncological screening with MRI: Opportunities, challenges and limitations

Heinz-Peter Schlemmer

11.1 Introduction

"The 21st century: The age of screening" is the title of a review published by Richard M. Friedberg from the Department of Radiological Science at the University of California in the journal "Radiology" in 2002 on the subject of radiological screening examinations [1]. This development is understandable considering that enormous technological progress in imaging techniques currently coincides with a transition in the understanding of disease. Enhanced health consciousness, a longer average lifespan, and increasing self-reliance, in part politically enforced, in matters concerning health and sickness in the enlightened and well informed population of the western world lead to this change in thinking. While in the past the healthcare system primarily concentrated on paying doctors to cure diseases whose symptoms had become evident and to provide all the medical and technical resources as far as possible, now more attention is demanded for the early diagnosis of chronic and incurable diseases. This raised health consciousness is now met with the ever-more impressive possibilities of radiological imaging for screening pathological changes. Understandably, a steadily growing commercial healthcare sector is developing in parallel in the economy.

Screening examinations have long since been propagated by politicians and investors in the healthcare system. For example, screening of colorectal carcinomas using the stool test and two coloscopies is offered as part of the catalog of benefits of the statutory health insurance funds in Germany since October 2002. There still appears to be a contradiction between the health consciousness among the population, which is also politically encouraged, on the one hand, and continuing discussions on the necessity of reducing medial expenditure, on the other. The impression is easily formed that the current preventive care opportunities are not being fully exploited. Demand for preventive examinations using whole-body magnetic resonance imaging (MRI) therefore usually comes not from doctors who should serve their patients as part of a preventive care concept, but more from the medical laymen or "self referrers" or "customers" who want to look after their own health by staying (more or less) informed through the media. However, the cost-benefit ratio of "incidental findings/secondary diagnoses" for examining healthy customers or asymptomatic patients depends on the individual therapeutic consequences and has yet to be clarified [2].

In the last 10 years, computed tomography (CT) has made great progress, so that whole-body examinations for oncological investigations have now become routine. This technological advancement also led to this type of preventive examination being offered commercially at an early stage in the USA. The use of X-rays in (supposedly) healthy people is however problematic for medical, ethical, as well as legal reasons. This is demonstrated by the continuing discussions surrounding the use of X-ray mammography in breast cancer screening. With the exception of X-ray mammography, the European Union has even banned the use of X-rays for the purposes of preventive examinations [3]. MRI, on the other hand, does not require ionizing radiation and also achieves a better soft tissue contrast, for example of the brain, the parenchymatous organs, and the bone marrow, which is decisive for oncological examinations. Interest in screening examinations using MRI is therefore high, despite the drawbacks of long examination times and high costs.

Whole-body MRI is still at a relatively early stage, but is nevertheless the imaging method of the future. Pioneering work on screening with whole-body MRI firstly built upon the technique of contrast-enhanced MR angiography of the whole body with a self-made movable patient platform [4]. Initial large-scale preventive examinations using whole-body MR angiography and virtual MR colonoscopy have already been performed [5–7]. Technological advancements now allow high-resolution whole-body MRI in a single examination procedure, also taking oncological considerations into account [8]. The development of modern whole-body MR technology has therefore fundamentally changed the discussion regarding MRI for oncological secondary prevention.

How, to what extent, and with which evidence cancer screening with whole-body MRI can be performed is not yet documented through studies. Although the development of methods is currently in a state of flux and the outcomes are open, a major medical potential is still recognizable. The following account should serve to cast a critical insight into this new and multifaceted field of modern radiology, which is sure to attain increasing importance in the future. Not only should the opportunities be discussed, but also the challenges, problems and limitations which provide or have provided the impetus for new research.

11.2 The concept of oncological prevention

The aim of prevention is to reduce the disease-specific mortality, i.e. to extend the lives of the group examined. Primary prevention (prophylaxis) and secondary prevention (screening) and tertiary prevention (countering the advancement of a disease) are methodologically distinguished.

The best-known example for successful preventive regulation is prophylaxis of caries and periodontosis according to the motto "prevention is better than cure". The aim of primary prevention is active prevention of the origin of a disease. Regular information and training on sensible nutrition, regular dental care, as well as preventive examinations paid by the health insurance funds have, combined with timely therapy, led to measurable successes in dental health in the population. Secondary prevention means regular check-up examinations of the teeth, which are themselves considered to be healthy, and tertiary prevention includes actions, e.g. regular dental check-ups and care of the gums in case of manifest periodontosis, to avoid or at least delay later complications, such as tooth loss. Addressing the benefit of preventive dental measures, there is no doubt that the financial investment of prevention is clearly balanced by the costs of treatment saved. It obviously not only makes medical sense, but is also economically favorable to visit the doctor "in a healthy state", as timely diagnosis and therefore treatment of diseased teeth is cheaper than the subsequent treatment at an advanced stage, where consequential damage and chronic problems require more elaborate measures of treatment. For this reason, regular dental preventive examinations and educational programs are carried out even in children's nursery schools.

There are however several problem areas when it comes to oncological screening measures, which have to be considered in a differentiated approach. Whereas in the primary prevention of cardiovascular disease changes in lifestyle, such as weight reduction, dietary changes, exercise, or stress reduction, are epidemiologically proven and are in principle practicable, such basic health enhancing changes in lifestyle are not sufficient for primary prevention of cancerous diseases. Until now, approaches towards primary prevention are only indicated if causal factors for the origin of the disease are known and may be excluded, e.g. refraining from smoking to avoid bronchial carcinoma. An established role of occupational medicine is the avoidance of carcinogenic substances or radiation at the workplace. However, for the most common tumors, such as breast and prostate carcinoma, as well as less common tumors, e.g. brain tumor and sarcomas, there are no scientifically proven factors influencing the origin of the disease. Carcinogenesis is a complex and multifactorial phenomenon.

Secondary and tertiary prevention therefore currently represent the most important approaches towards reducing cancer-related mortality. The aim of secondary prevention measures is a diagnosis as early as possible in case of the existing, but not yet symptomatic disease, i.e. before the patient consults the doctor with symptoms. Tertiary prevention finally serves to prevent or at least delay the advancement of the tumor disease and its complications by performing regular follow-up examinations. Alongside the medical history, clinical and laboratory chemical investigations, imaging diagnostics play an essential role in secondary and tertiary prevention of cancerous disease. It must still be borne in mind that in whole-body MRI tumor screening, the boundaries between secondary (early diagnosis) and tertiary prevention (follow-up care) may be blurred. In contrast to the determination of a specific tumor marker (e.g. PSA), whole-body MRI is a broad-based and unspecifically directed method. For this reason, secondary prevention can include one tumor entity (e.g. colorectal carcinoma) and tertiary prevention can include another (e.g. mamma carcinoma 10 years ago). Those who have personally decided to have a cancer screening examination may have a medical history with a high family risk for the development of a tumor disease or may have even already suffered one.

To examine all persons for all conceivable tumor diseases is, of course, neither medically nor economically viable. The efficiency of dental preventive measures, on the other hand, is quite obvious and is attributable to four reasons: 1. The prevalence of caries and periodontosis is extremely high in our society, so that retrospectively a preventive examination is justified in many cases. 2. The early stage of dental disease can be ascertained in a timely manner, as the disease generally starts on the tooth surface. 3. Diagnosis of the disease at an early stage is possible with a high degree of accuracy with a cheap and harmless examination method, namely the inspection of the tooth and in individual cases a supplementary X-ray examination. 4. An effective therapy is uncomplicated for the dentist to perform. These four points correspond precisely to the four criteria Wilson and Junger stated in 1968 as being necessary for effective screening for a specific disease: a) high prevalence of the disease, b) detectability at an early stage, c) existence of an effective examination method, and d) ability to perform an effective therapy [9].

The following considerations therefore arise in regard to developing viable strategies for effective tumor prevention using whole-body MRI:

ad 1. Prevalence: Carcinogenesis is, as previously mentioned, a complex and multifactorial phenomenon and is not uniform for different tumor entities. Some causal risk factors have been proven, e.g. smoking, alcohol consumption, or special dietary habits. The greatest risk factor for the origin of cancer, however, is age. Against the background of the over-aging society, an increase in the frequency of cancer must be anticipated. The further increase in cancer mortality is also to be expected in the western world, because the mortality from cardiovascular disease has significantly dropped over the last three decades. The large and heterogeneous group of cancer diseases, however, encompasses a multitude of diseases with widely varying prevalence. The most common malignant tumors include the bronchial, mamma, prostate, and colorectal carcinoma with a fatality of around 10–25%. Less common malignant tumors are those of the ovaries, stomach, pancreas, kidneys, and bladder, whose fatality is in the range 3–6%. A detailed list of the frequency of tumors in Germany is to be found in the cancer registry [10].

If the prevalence of the disease among the group of persons examined is higher than in a random cross-section of the population, the examination will more probably discover positive results and will therefore be more efficient. Precise preselection into certain risk groups is therefore desirable. An accompanying general/internal medicine examination and consultation should therefore be an integral part of the preventive examination.

For the individual, the identification of risk factors can provide an argument for having the preventive examination performed. From a statistical viewpoint, the examination of a high-risk group would definitely be more efficient than that of the entire collective. However, efficiency considerations are of no significance for the individual, as the absence of these risk factors does not exclude the presence of the disease with any certainty. The measured frequency of discovered tumors also depends on the examination method applied. The advancements in MR technology have recently facilitated the performance of a whole-body MRI in "state-of-the-art" quality for individual regions of the body, which promises an increase in the effectiveness of the whole-body examination.

ad 2. Detectability at an early stage: In principle, many solid and hematological tumor entities can be discovered at an early stage even without the use of MRI, such as colorectal carcinomas using coloscopy or the malignant melanoma through dermatological inspection. On the other hand, in the case of rapidly proliferating tumors, early diagnosis considerations at the presymptomatic stage are questionable or even hopeless, as in the case of acute leukemia. It is difficult to define from which age onwards which tumor entities should be searched for with MRI and at which intervals.

The time for the initial diagnosis and the subsequent early diagnosis intervals have to be oriented towards the biological activity, i.e. the growth rate, of the respective tumor entity. The growth patterns of tumors is however extremely variable and is also dependent on individual factors and is therefore hard to predict in the individual case. The faster and more aggressive the tumor grows, the shorter the check-up intervals should be. Mamma carcinoma, for example, is generally a faster and more aggressively growing tumor than prostate carcinoma. Dependent upon the tumor entity observed, an examination interval selected too long increases the rate of tumors originating and consequently not being detected in the interval, whereas, conversely, an interval selected too short leads to ineffectiveness and unnecessary stress for the person examined. The age-related incidence of tumors also indicates that the prevention interval should be adapted to age. Concerning this point, prostate carcinoma screening examinations were for example performed using PSA screening [11]: A cohort of 17,226 men aged between 55 and 74 years were randomized and divided into two groups, an intervention and a control group. The intervention group had a PSA value determination in serum performed before and after a 4-year interval. Both groups received a common standard treatment from a private urologist, independent of the study. In the 4-year interval, 18 unpredicted carcinomas were detected in the screening group and 135 carcinomas in the control group, which corresponds to a relative rate of so-called "interval carcinomas" of around 13% in the intervention or screening group. Also, the tumors found in the screening group during the interval were all in an organ-limited stage. The sensitivity of the screening was 85.5% overall. The authors therefore conclude that a 4-year control interval for PSA screening of men between 55 and 74 years is appropriate. Similar studies generally need to be made available for other tumor entities and for whole-body MRI.

ad 3. Effective examination method: The examination method must allow the detection of the disease in its early stage. In general, there is a broad and highly efficient range of laboratory and imaging examination methods available, which allow precise diagnosis of tumor diseases at an early stage. On the other hand, it must be borne in mind that all examination techniques are also associated with risks: Firstly, there exists the obvious risk of method-related morbidity, e.g. as a consequence of intravenous administration of contrast agent. Secondly, an at first less apparent but possibly even graver risk exists that, in the case of a false-positive or false-negative result and the related unnecessary or inappropriate treatment, morbidity and mortality can ensue. For example, the radiological diagnosis of a suspected tumor can give rise to repeated biopsies or an operation, which, if the result is retrospectively ascertained as false-positive, has led to superfluous physical and possibly psychological damage to a healthy person. An example of a problem evaluated in depth is the early diagnosis of a prostate carcinoma by means of determining the prostate-specific antigen (PSA) in serum [12]. On the one hand, PSA is one of the best and also most conclusive serum markers for early diagnosis of a tumor; on the other hand, PSA increases can also be caused by benign diseases of the prostate, e.g. through benign prostatic hypertrophy. Hence, the danger exists that men are subjected to unnecessary biopsies and live with the fear of having a tumor disease. And even if prostate carcinoma is discovered, there is still nothing known about the aggressivity of the disease, which is well known to be biologically very variable, i.e. whether the tumor would ever have led to symptoms during the lifetime of the patient. The old medical principle "nil nocere" should receive consideration.

Experience from breast cancer screening using X-ray mammography has shown that the best possible preventive examinations at a high technical level can only be performed by specially trained and experienced radiologists. It has also been shown that the reliability of the diagnosis can be increased by double reading by two independent radiologists. In the case of breast cancer screening, the medical and economic advantages achieved by setting up specialized and quality-controlled centers have become obvious.

ad 4. Effective therapy: The therapy concepts for tumor diseases are very complex, subject to continuous change, and are therefore no longer manageable for the individual doctor. Interdisciplinary therapy strategies adapted to studies and defined according to the individual condition, including surgery, chemotherapy, radiation therapy, and their combination in adjuvant and neoadjuvant treatment concepts, render interdisciplinary cooperation necessary. For many cancerous diseases, therapeutic success crucially depends on the tumor stage in the initial diagnosis. Also, the cause of death for most types of tumors is not the local tumor but rather distant metastasis. The preventive examination is targeted at the early diagnosis of the tumor disease at the stage of exclusively local extension. The probability of metastasis is not necessarily, but still frequently, linked with the tumor size. In the symptomatic stage, there is unfortunately often an advanced tumor stage. The aim of early diagnosis has to be to catch the tumor disease in the presymptomatic stage, where the probability of metastasis is still low. The rationale for the preventive examination is that treatment with the means available today is generally more promising the earlier the diagnosis is made. An example is X-ray mammography for early diagnosis of breast cancer. Data have been gathered in clinical studies over the past 40 years or so, and there conclusiveness has been discussed extremely controversially and relentlessly. It can be justifiably claimed that X-ray mammography is the most precisely investigated imaging technique for the early diagnosis of cancer and therefore provides important insights with respect to tumor prevention based on imaging techniques [13].

11.3 The role of MRI in oncological early diagnosis

The measurable efficiency of a preventive examination depends on both the prevalence of the disease in the group studied, as well as the accuracy of the examination method. According to experience, besides optimizing the examination protocols, only through targeted preselection of a certain risk group (e.g. family risk for the occurrence of a colorectal carcinoma) can an increase in efficiency of the examination method be achieved.

The efficiency of preventive examination methods cannot be determined on the basis of small studies. Nevertheless, irrespective of these considerations, tumors discovered in the early and therefore possibly curable stage, whether as "secondary results" from a dedicated MRI or as part of a preventive examination, can be of great importance for the individual. For the person affected, the general cost efficiency of the method is then insignificant. An example from personal experience is the discovery of a bladder carcinoma in the presymptomatic stage, which could be treated simply by cystoscopic removal and with a good prognosis. At the symptomatic stage there may well have been growth through the wall that would have required a cystectomy, and the prognosis would have been severely impaired. It is still clear, however, that general screening of the population for bladder tumors is not cost efficient on account of their low incidence. The debate surrounding preventive examinations using whole-body MRI is unavoidably subject to the conflicting priorities of individual impact and cost efficiency. The following account looks at the proven role of MRI in screening the most frequently occurring tumors in the western world.

11.3.1 Bronchial carcinoma

The bronchial carcinoma (BC) is currently the most common fatal tumor in the western world. With respect to cancer mortality, the bronchial carcinoma is the most common tumor among men and the third most common tumor among women. Although the frequency among women is on the rise due to the increased number of female smokers, it is in slow decline among men. The tumor often only becomes symptomatic in the advanced stage in which the average 5-year survival rate is below 15%.

As in tuberculosis screening, conventional X-ray images are firstly taken for early diagnosis of bronchial carcinoma and sputum investigations are used. The use of CT enables smaller tumors in the presymptomatic stage to be discovered [14]. Even though it is acknowledged that earlier stages of BC can be discovered by CT, it is disputed whether mortality can be reduced as a result. Initial results of randomized studies will soon be available. An extensive discussion is presented on the problem of lung cancer screening by the Henschke work group [15].

A problem in preventive examination with CT is that by far not all coin lesions discovered are also malignant. But the detection of coin lesions in many cases compels control examinations, which according to current research knowledge should be performed with CT every 12 months for diameters of less than 5 mm and every 3 months if larger than 5 mm. It has to be considered that the examinations are associated with radiation exposure each time. Outside of studies, radiological lung cancer screening is not recommended at present [17].

The examination of the lungs is clearly a domain of conventional X-ray and CT. MRI is of no importance in routine diagnostics of BC, which could however change in the near future in the light of the rapid pace of technological development. Studies published so far on the diagnostics of coin lesions using MRI already show that the sensitivity from a lesion size of 5 mm upwards is around 90% compared with CT [18–19]. Whether the analysis of signal intensities of coin lesions with T1 and T2-weighted sequences or contrast agent dynamics can reveal information on their benignity is the subject of ongoing research [19–20].

11.3.2 Colorectal carcinoma

The colorectal carcinoma is in second place in the statistics for tumor-related causes of death for both genders [10]. Secondary prevention of colorectal carcinoma is worthwhile, as the development usually takes place with long latency (approx. 10 years) from adenomas, and an endoscopic polypectomy is easy to perform as therapy [21–22]. Conventional optical colonoscopy can be performed for detection, or virtual colonoscopy using CT (CTC) or MRI (MRC). CTC data are available from a large study with 1233 asymptomatic participants [23], which showed a high accuracy compared with colonoscopy (sensitivity of 89–94% dependent on the polyp size). Initial results with MRC in smaller study collectives indicate that this method can also be used to find clinically relevant polyps with diameters ≥10 mm with the same detection rate [24]. The advantage of MRC over CTC is primarily the absence of radiation exposure, which allows both dynamic examinations of the bowl after i.v. contrast media administration to analyze polyp perfusion, as well as examinations of other regions of the body as part of whole-body tumor prevention. Through the use of parallel imaging, examination times can be reduced such that a virtual MR colonoscopy can easily be integrated into the overall examination protocol. The customer/patient examined must definitely be informed, however, that no adequate data are available in the literature to document the effectiveness of MR colonoscopy for early diagnosis of colorectal polyps.

11.3.3 Breast carcinoma

Breast carcinoma is the most common cancerous disease for women, presents an aggressive biological development, and in its advanced stage is connected with high mortality. The diagnostic strategies are clearly defined in the guidelines of the German Society of Senology [25]. Early diagnosis of mamma carcinoma using mammography has been performed and studied for around 40 years, but the discussion of its benefit is still very controversial. Development is very slow in achieving an evidence-based knowledge base in this complex area that would bring about a unified approach towards regulated preventive examinations.

The performance of a dedicated MR mammography with high local resolution and contrast agent dynamics as part of whole-body MRI is not possible for practical reasons. In addition, on account of its low positive predictive value, MR mammography is not generally recommended for primary diagnostics of breast carcinoma. Exceptions are high-risk patients with enlarged gland parenchyma, for whom screening with MR mammography is viewed as being indicated [26]. This dynamic examination after administration of i.v. contrast agent cannot however be usefully integrated into the concept of a whole-body examination.

It is to be expected with whole-body MRI that due to the high prevalence of both benign and malignant findings in the female breast, especially in premenopausal women, several mamma lesions will be detected that cannot be classified with certainty due to inadequate specificity. In advance of the examination, the patient/customer should be informed that no tumor prediction in regard to mamma carcinoma is possible by means of whole-body MRI, and that in the case of detected lesions in the mamma, their reliable assessment may not be possible. In this case further treatment, firstly through the gynecologist, must take place for adequate classification, which includes common conventional diagnostics with mammography and ultrasound as necessary. In the case of larger lesions, a subsequent MR mammographic clarification may be worthwhile, as in this case a high specificity is to be expected on account of the morphology of the lesion [27]. Patients must always be informed about the lack of specificity and the inadequate sensitivity of the method for breast carcinoma screening prior to a whole-body MRI, and this should be documented in writing.

11.3.4 Prostate carcinoma

Prostate carcinoma is the most common carcinoma after bronchial carcinoma and the second most frequent male malignant tumor disease leading to death. There are around 31,500 men in Germany alone who suffer a prostate carcinoma per year, and around 11,000 men die of it in the same period [10]. Since the 1980s, the introduction of a simple PSA serum test has made an essential contribution to early diagnosis with tumor propagation often still limited to the prostate. In this respect, the effectiveness of the test has been documented in a large randomized study. The evidence of reduction in mortality is still unproven, however [28–29]. Here the results of the PLCO trials, for example, are to be awaited [30]. Further advancements in the PSA test, e.g. the determination of the ratio of free to total PSA, are promising and are currently under investigation.

Transrectal ultrasound (TRUS) is still considered to be the first imaging modality in the case of suspected prostate carcinoma and is used for image-controlled biopsy. The major importance of MRI with combined endorectal and body-phased array coils (endo MRI) is undisputed for local staging of histologically proven prostate carcinoma. Following bioptic diagnosis, organ specific tumor growth can be distinguished from tumor growth transgressing the organ and/or infiltrating the seminal vesicles with high specificity (up to approx. 90%), which yields important information to decide on the individual therapy strategy. MRI is also without doubt the most sensitive method (approx. 90%) currently available with the highest spatial resolution. The low specificity (approx. 50%) is nevertheless a problem which impairs differential diagnosis towards prostatitis and benign prostate hypertrophy (BPH) even in the case of an identified increase in PSE serum concentration. The measurement of MRI-based PSA density could enhance specificity [31].

A T2-weighted MRI of the pelvis should be performed as part of the preventive examination. The combination of high sensitivity with concomitant low specificity is however very problematic for the diagnosis of the prostate. The use of an endorectal coil to improve the spatial resolution is not feasible for whole-body MRI due to the long examination time, but is also not useful as the specificity of the method is not fundamentally improved as a result. The examination usually entails detection of diverse, but not clearly classifiable, pathological signal changes of the prostate, because in the age group examined, the incidence of both benign changes of the prostate, such as BPH and various forms of prostatitis, as well as prostate carcinoma, is high. Dynamic, contrast-enhanced MRI and [1]H-MR spectroscopic imaging have the potential to better differentiate malignant from benign changes and therefore improve the diagnostic accuracy of MRI [32–33]. A dedicated MRI examination using the endorectal coil is however obligatory here. The importance of MRI for early diagnostics could above all be to more precisely localize regions of suspected carcinoma in the case of a PSA increase and therefore provide an indication for biopsy, but there are insufficient data available at present. These methods are also not to be performed as part of a preventive examination using whole-body MRI.

As part of whole-body MRI, it should be discussed with the customer/patient that an adequate accuracy for early diagnosis of prostate carcinoma is not possible. A supplementary preventive urological examination is recommended in this regard. Information as to the limited conclusiveness of the method in regard to the detection of prostate carcinoma should be documented in every case. If a suspicious result is found with MR imaging and urological tests are also available in which a prostate carcinoma is suspected, the supplementary performance of MRI with endorectal coil, as described above, can be discussed.

11.3.5 Less common tumors

MRI offers, for example, high accuracy in the detection and differential diagnosis of ovarian processes; effective preventive care of ovarian carcinoma is also possible with a combination of transvaginal ultrasound and the determination of the CA-125 marker [34]. In the detection of pancreas carcinoma, CT and MRI show comparable sensitivities of 70 to 80% [35]. The importance of MRI in the early diagnosis and staging of stomach carcinoma for instance is still completely unclear [36]. Preventive care with regard to renal cell carcinoma can in principle be performed with ultrasound [37], although this examination is in turn limited as compared with MRI in respect to the diagnostics of other organs. The potential of MRI as an initial method for early diagnosis of less common tumors, such as renal cell or pancreas carcinoma, is still uncertain. In this regard, the results of smaller studies and experience in daily clinical radiological practice with incidentally discovered tumors have to be drawn upon. Renal cell carcinomas can certainly be detected with high sensitivity in their early stages using MRI. MRI also offers high accuracy (over 90%) in the differential diagnosis of ovarian processes [34]. The importance of MRI, for instance for early diagnosis of stomach carcinoma, is currently the subject of scientific investigation [36, 38]. Possible special investigative methods, such as distension of the stomach, are hardly feasible to perform within the scope of a whole-body examination. The performance of conventional gastroscopy is required for early diagnosis of stomach carcinoma. The general diagnostic algorithm for early diagnosis is not clearly defined for most tumors and is also in a state of flux. Advances in MR technology mean that changes in approach are to be expected.

11.4 Whole-body magnetic resonance imaging for oncological screening

11.4.1 Examination protocols and data evaluation

A "state of the art" MRI of a region of the body requires the use of a surface coil. In order to examine more than one region of the body, e.g. the brain and the abdomen, it was therefore necessary for technical reasons to reposition the patient with the appropriate change of coils. An optimal whole-body examination was therefore impracticable until recently. The optimal administration of intravenous contrast agent in a single examination procedure was also not possible due to the necessary repositioning of the patient and the resulting time delay. The first whole-body examinations were carried out with table movement and the use of the whole-body coil [39] or a phase array coil (Angio*SURF*®) [40–41]. The second technique has already been applied for screening cardiovascular diseases, and a MR colonoscopy was integrated for the detection of colorectal polyps [5–7].

Technical advancements in the field of coil technology and parallel imaging now facilitate the high-resolution presentation of the entire body in a single examination using state-of-the-art technology [8]. A new 1.5 Tesla system allows the connection of up to 76 coil elements and the synchronous acquisition of up to 32 independent receiver channels (MAGNETOM Avanto, Siemens Medical Solutions, Erlangen, Germany). In combination with automatic table movement, 500 mm field of view, a high performance gradient system (max. amplitude: 45 mT/m), and parallel imaging in all three spatial planes, high-resolution whole-body MRI can be performed with a maximum examination length of 205 cm in just under one hour. Patients are placed in a supine position with arms positioned alongside the body. Dependent on the body size, a total of 5–6 phased array coils with several individual coil elements are used: 12 coil elements for the head, 4 for the neck, 6 each for the thorax, abdomen and pelvis, 16 for the low extremities, and 24 elements embedded in the table for the spinal column. Positioning the coils takes around 3 min. Experience so far indicates that the use of a large number of surface coils does not induce claustrophobia in the patients.

A typical oncological screening examination protocol with the new multi-channel system, which was installed in the Radiological University Clinic in Tübingen, Germany, in November 2003, is presented in the following. The examination protocol has been applied at the University of Tübingen both for secondary prevention without clinical evidence for cancerous disease, as well as in a slightly modified version for tertiary prevention and metastasis search given the presence of a cancerous disease [8, 42]. The performance, i.e. practicability and efficiency of the whole-body MRI for metastasis search, was investigated in a collective of patients with advanced melanoma (stage III and IV) in comparison with whole-body CT [43]. This study showed that the result of the whole-body MRI led to a change in the therapeutic concept in approx. 25% of the patients examined.

This is essentially due to the higher sensitivity of MRI in the detection of 1. cerebral, 2. hepatic, and 3. bone metastasis (bone marrow carcinosis without bone decomposition). The results also led to prompt acceptance of the examination from the referring physicians, as well as from patients informed via various sources who have to act as "self referrers", as the insurance companies do not offer a billing code for whole-body MRI.

The measurements are generally performed at 5 different table positions, and standard MR examination protocols can, in principle, be arbitrarily combined with one another

(Table 11.1). Experience with whole-body MRI based on TIRM (Short Tau Inversion Recovery) sequences is already available [44–47]. A coronal STIR turbo spin-echo (TSE) sequence is therefore preferably performed at the beginning of the examination and serves to examine the bone marrow. The additionally integrated examination modules include axial FLAIR (Fluid Attenuated Inversion Recovery) and T1w-SE sequences for the head; axial TIRM and VIBE (Volume Interpolated Breath-hold Examination) sequences for the thorax; and axial fat-saturated T2w-TSE and T1w-SE sequences for the abdomen. The fat-saturated T2w-TSE sequence for the abdomen is carried out with a navigator under free breathing conditions; the other examinations of the thorax and abdomen are performed in breath-hold. Examination of the spinal column entails sagittal STIR or T2w-TSE sequences, which are supplemented with axial T2w-TSE sequences depending on the result. Magnetic resonance colonoscopy (MRC) is performed after repositioning the patient. The "dark lumen"

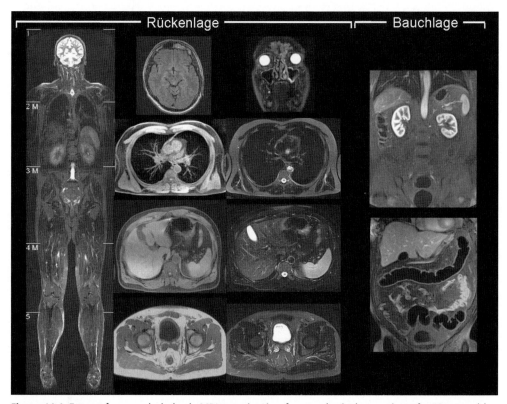

Figure 11.1 Extract from a whole-body MRI examination for oncological screening of a 53-year-old man with history of an inverted papilloma. The patient was also a smoker. On the left is the coronal STIR image of the whole body. Presented in the center is the axial FLAIR image (left) and coronal STIR image of the skull, as well as axial T1-weighted (left) and T2-weighted (right) images of the thorax, abdomen and pelvis. Coronal VIBE images following i.v. administration of Gd-DTPA in the arterial (top) and portal venous (bottom) phases. The examination protocol is listed in Table 11.1. A soft tissue mass in the sinus ethmoidalis and frontalis left was found, leading to the suspicion of recurrence of the inverted papilloma in its presymptomatic stage. (From: Schäfer JF, Fischmann A, Lichy M, Vollmar J, Fenchel M, Claussen CD, Schlemmer HP. Der Radiologe 2004; 44: 854–863, with kind permission of Springer Verlag)

Table 11.1 Typical examination protocol for oncological screening using whole-body MRI

Region of the body	Orien-tation	Weighting/ sequence type	TR/TE/TI (ms/ms/ms)	Section thickness – voxel size (mm)	Acquisition time [min]
Whole-body – head/neck – thorax/ abdomen – pelvis/prox. thigh – prox. thigh/dist. lower leg – dist. lower leg/feet	coronal	T2w STIR	 5490/87/150 6100/87/150 8540/87/150 7630/87/150 7380/87/150	5.0–1.8 × 1.3	Total = 11:48 2:44 3:04 2:17 2:02 1:43
Skull	axial	T1w SE FLAIR	500/8/- 9380/108/2500	4.0–0.9 × 0.9 1,2–0.9 × 0.9	2:59 2:30
Neck	axial	T1w FLASH 2D T2w-STIR	337/4.1/- 5560/59/150	5.0–1.1 × 0.8 5.0–1.2 × 0.9	0:48 2:17
Thorax	axial	T2w-STIR 3D VIBE fs	3800/100/150 3.37/1.21	6.0–1.8 × 1.2 2.0–2.0 × 2.0	0:48 (mbh) 0:20ˣ2 (bh)
Abdomen	axial	T1w FLASH 2D fs T2w TSE fs	242/4.1/- 5640/95/-	6.0–2.1 × 1.5 6.0–1.6 × 1.2	0:59 (mbh) ≈ 1:50 (rg)
Pelvis	axial	T1w FLASH 2D T2w STIR	248/4.1/- 7100/70/150	4.0–2.1 × 1.5 4.0–1.3 × 1.0	0:57 4:31
Abdomen and pelvis including MRC	coronal	3D VIBE fs	3.1/1.2/-	2.0 × 2.0 × 2.0	0:20 × 4[1] (bh)

STIR = Short Tau Inversion Recovery; fs = fat saturated; bh = breath-hold; mbh = multiple breath-hold; rg = respiratory gated; MRC = MR colonoscopy
[1] dynamic MRI with 1 measurement before and 3 measurements after administration of i.v. CA

technique is performed, following an enema of around 1.5–2 l of body temperature tap water, by means of a VIBE sequence in hypotension (i.v. scopolamine) and with intravenous application of a paramagnetic contrast agent. Finally, T1-weighted axial images of the trunk (thorax/abdomen/pelvis) are produced. A typical examination protocol is specified in more detail in Table 11.1 and is illustrated in Figure 11.1. The complete examination protocol requires around 60 min; the approximate in-room time required including repositioning and enteroclysma is around 1.5 h. The time requirement for evaluation, documentation, and discussion of the complete image material is very variable and can take up to around 30–60 min.

11.4.2 Patient information and post-examination consultation

The consultation following oncological screening differs from consultations normally held by radiologists as part of their medical practice. The expectations of the customers/patients paying for the examination themselves are quite different from those referred for examination of a targeted part of the body to clarify a specific medical question (e.g. r/o meniscal tear?). The customers/patients generally take a great deal of time for the screening examination and tend to devote serious thought to their previous lifestyle. Not only the opportunities, but also the limitations of the examination method have to be explained to the customer/patient in advance of the examination. The possibility of false-positive and false-negative results must be pointed out in particular, as well as their consequences, which are easily underestimated by the medical layman on account of the impressive MR technology.

1. The outcome of a *true-negative result* is, of course, hoped for by the examinee as well as by the radiologist. But even if this is the case, it should be mentioned that this does not exclude the future origin of a tumor, because the momentary sense of security of the examinee can lead to future medical checkups with the primary care physician, gynecologist, urologist, etc. being neglected, which in turn leads to an increased risk for later diagnoses. The sense of security in the case of a negative result (e.g. no pulmonary mass lesion) can also cause a drop in motivation to cease a hazardous habit (e.g. smoking), thereby even deterring a positive change in lifestyle. For this reason, the post-examination consultation should include a survey of risk factors and should expressly indicate that irrespective of the outcome of the screening examination, all risk factors which can be influenced should be corrected and regular examinations should continue to be performed in the future. The question of whether, and at which intervals, whole-body MRI should be repeated is one that cannot be currently answered.

2. In the case of a *true-positive result,* it is hoped that the early diagnosis of the cancerous disease leads to a cure or at least to an improvement in life expectancy.
   This possible examination outcome is indeed feared, but it is the real reason why the screening examination was carried out in the first place. The conviction is, of course, that tumors discovered at an early stage, and therefore of smaller size, can generally be better treated. It is however little known that this does not apply to all tumor types, and that early diagnosis may only prolong the period of knowledge of the disease without actually extending life expectancy ("lead time bias", see below). On the other hand, for less aggressive tumors and for persons of advanced age, it cannot be certain whether the disease would ever have become symptomatic or even life limiting ("pseudo disease", see below). This problem has been e.g. discussed in the context of early diagnosis of prostate carcinoma, but is now also being discussed in the case of bronchial carcinoma. There is therefore the possibility that the screening examination with the diagnosis it reveals could actually impair life quality.

3. *A false-negative result* can either be unavoidable (method-related limitation in sensitivity and/or specificity) or avoidable (inadequate examination protocol, overlooked result). Lulling the customer/patient into a false sense of security can mean that newly occurring or even existing symptoms can be overlooked, thereby delaying the definitive diagnosis.

4. *False-positive results* can be seen retrospectively as having led to superfluous pain and psychological suffering of the examinee. It is additionally problematic that the consequential costs of supplementary examinations, unnecessary therapies with their associated morbidity/mortality, and labor absenteeism have to be borne by the general public, in contrast to the screening examination. All these factors lead to ethical problems and will have to be considered in the case of a lawsuit.

Consultation on the results and advice upon completion of the screening examination is generally open-ended and therefore demands a relatively long time: Firstly, it is naturally expected that the images are presented in general terms with an explanation of anatomical details and any findings, regardless of whether these are medically irrelevant (e.g. hemangioma), possibly require treatment (e.g. intervertebral disc protrusion), or are definitely relevant to therapy (e.g. suspicion of renal cell carcinoma). Depending on the interests of the person examined, even the first viewing of the images can develop into a small anatomy course for beginners. For all the results found (also non-oncological secondary results, such as intervertebral disc protrusion), advice is obviously expected in regard to possible therapies or preventive measures. This is sensible, as the screening examination is only considered to be useful in retrospect if the examination results are also followed with specific consequences. Furthermore, open questions usually arise from the consultation concerning the individual options for primary prevention, i.e. advice is expected as to how, and through which changes in lifestyle, a contribution can be made towards an individual preventive program in general and cancer prevention in particular. Consultations of this type can easily overstretch the radiologist, not only in terms of their available time but also specialist competence. It is also to be borne in mind that the mere mention of the suspicion of a cancerous disease can cause severe psychological stress for the person affected, as well as for their relatives. If a malignant result really has been found, a concept for the further diagnostic and therapeutic approach should also be available very quickly. Prior to whole-body MRI it should already be thought out who is to continue care for the customer/patient in case there is a result pointing to a tumor. Because, at this moment, the customer/patient is understandably confronted with a flood of notions, expectations, and fears concerning further examinations, possible operations, chemotherapy, or radiation therapy. All this has to be covered in a medical consultation, so that the patient leaves the radiologist with a clear understanding of the subsequent approach. The integration of the examination into a well thought-out and planned concept for the subsequent medical care is also to be encouraged from an ethical perspective.

11.5 Cost-efficiency considerations

The key question, and, at the same time, the crux of public debate on the pros and cons of early diagnosis measures, is whether the health advantages balance with their risks and costs. The discussion is generally conducted under the premise that the advantages and risks of the screening examination affect the patient, whereas the costs are borne by the general public. Two different perspectives are in conflict: the perspective of the individual, who wants the best done for his/her health, and the perspective of the health insurance companies that have to responsibly budget the funds available to them and only pay for early diagnosis if this leads to an overall drop in morbidity or mortality. For the health insurance companies, the aim of prevention is balanced by the expenditure required, i.e. the money ultimately required for it. The efficiency of screening examinations is checked on the grounds of a cost-benefit analysis and is quantified in costs per life year gained. Reliable data on cost-efficiency can only be obtained from randomized studies for which a representative part of the population is prospectively and randomly allocated to two groups with and without a screening examination and by comparing their mortality.

Statistically well-designed and conclusive studies without systematic error or bias are, however, generally very complex, laborious, and therefore expensive. For the correct planning of a prospective study, several influencing factors must be taken into consideration for statistical reasons, which are largely independent of the method actually tested (e.g. MR colonoscopy). These include the prospective definition of the study population and of the study period to obtain a particular level of statistical significance, the correct blinded randomization of the study participants, and the binding decision at the outset of the study for a defined end point both in terms of the measurement parameter (e.g. disease-related survival), as well as the point in time of data evaluation (e.g. after 10 years). Moreover, it has to be clarified how sources of error, which possibly occur during the course of the study but are unavoidable, are to be handled, for example if study participants rescind on the initial agreement and either demand ("contamination") or refuse ("non-compliance") the method under investigation (e.g. MR colonoscopy).

If the measurement results of the study are available at the end of the defined study period, then careful interpretation of the date is required. When evaluating the data in regard to disease-specific mortality, it must be precisely analyzed whether other causes of death have also arisen within the study period which could distort the evaluation results. The interpretation of results of clinical studies can also be distorted by several systematic faults in the study design (bias). These sources of error should be investigated at the outset of the study for the correct planning of the study design. The results and interpretations of previously published studies should also be critically assessed. The most important sources of error in randomized studies are the following:

1. "Selection bias": The structure of the participants of an oncological screening study can be one-sided in that persons with existing risk tend to want to participate, e.g. those with raised incidence of cancerous diseases in the family.
2. "Lead time bias": The early diagnosis of a cancerous disease shifts the time of the initial diagnosis, whereas the time of death could remain unchanged. Only the calculated survival time after the diagnosis is made is extended as a result, but not the actual lifetime. In this case, the early diagnosis measure has only extended the period of the identified disease, but has only apparently prolonged survival. The prolonged period of disease might even have caused the life quality of the patient to have been impaired over a longer period.
3. "Over-diagnosis" or "pseudo-disease": How a cancerous disease detected in the early stage develops can often only be conjectured but never known with certainty. The rationale for a tumor therapy is that the tumor will develop into a life threatening disease in the foreseeable future. This is not necessarily the case on an individual basis, and the disease might not have become apparent during the lifetime of the patient. In this case, the therapy of the disease, which would never have become symptomatic in the lifetime, leads only to an apparent therapeutic success. The patient would have received the label of a "pseudo-disease" through the early diagnosis. This difficulty arises for example in the discussion on the early diagnosis of prostate carcinoma.
4. "Length bias sampling": Screening examinations carried out regularly tend to discover slower rather than faster growing tumors, because, in the case of the latter, there is a higher probability that symptoms appear in the interval between the screening examinations. Retrospectively, the prognosis appears better for tumors discovered by the screening examination.

The following conclusions must be drawn and critically discussed from the data: How can sensitivity and specificity of the examination method be optimally balanced with one another and how is the resulting so-called "intervention threshold" to be defined? How many false-positive or false-negative results are to be accepted and how much superfluous therapeutic intervention must be necessarily tolerated in retrospect. How should the screening intervals be defined for future examinations? Taking the example of MR colonoscopy, the following specific questions arise for instance, which can only be answered with studies with a correct statistical design: With which accuracy (dependent on the method) can colorectal polyps be identified above a certain size? From what size of colorectal polyp found should a conventional colonoscopic, histological clarification be induced and up to what size is progress monitoring recommended? In which intervals do control examinations have to be performed to avoid numerous aggressively growing tumors being overlooked?

The worldwide largest controlled and randomized study on oncological prevention performed to date is the PLCO (Prostate, Lung, Colon, Ovarian) Cancer Screening Trial with a total number of almost 155,000 participants [30]. Whole-body MRI for imaging diagnostics was not available for consideration at the start of the trial, and only X-ray examinations of the thorax and transvaginal ultrasound examinations were performed. With regard to the importance of MRI in early diagnosis, there are still no results of randomized studies available, even for the most commonly occurring tumors, such as bronchial or colorectal carcinoma.

11.6 Summary and outlook

Rapid developments in MR technology have enabled whole-body MRI to be performed without difficulty within one single examination procedure. But even for the most common cancerous diseases, the potential of MRI in oncological screening is still being investigated in scientific studies and is therefore not yet reliably documented. The greatest wealth of experience is currently available on screening for colorectal carcinoma by means of virtual MR colonoscopy; the importance of MRI for bronchial carcinoma is still unclear, and there is currently no indication for breast and prostate carcinoma. On the other hand, experience has shown that uncommon cancerous diseases can also be discovered with whole-body MRI in the presymptomatic early stage and can then be treated with a very good prognosis and without therapy-related morbidity. An example is given of the incidental detection of a cystic meningioma, still asymptomatic at the time of the screening examination, which would probably however have become symptomatic in the near future due to its volume displacing aspect, e.g. in the form of a seizure (Fig. 11.2). The early diagnosis at the asymptomatic stage was able to prevent possible subsequent complications, possibly of a secondary cause, e.g. due to an accident resulting from a seizure. There are still no data from randomized studies to document the cost-efficiency of whole-body MRI. And until evidence is forthcoming that the examination also actually reduces expenditure on therapy and aftercare, the method cannot yet be recommended for oncological prevention in terms of health economics. Nonetheless, as the above example shows, the unexpected early diagnosis of a tumor can be of major importance to the individual affected, and the term "cost-efficiency" is of no relevance to the person affected at this moment. The discussion of the pros and cons of oncological screening examinations using whole-body MRI must also be controversially continued from two widely differing perspectives: On the one hand, the customer/patient can use the potential of modern MRI for his/her own personal prevention; on the other, the health insurance companies must budget their available funds to finance all medical services. The radiologist with his/her medical responsibility therefore stands in the middle of the conflict between what they can best offer the individual medi-

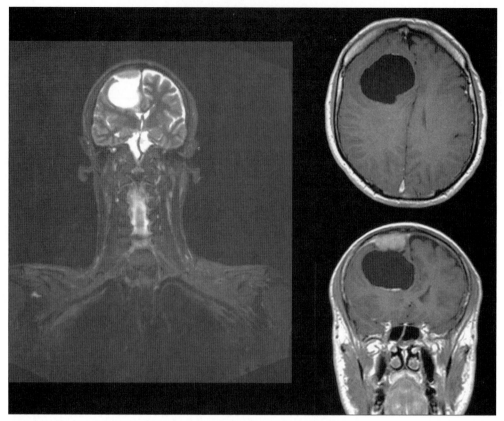

Figure 11.2 Part of a whole-body MRI examination of a non-symptomatic 47-year-old-man who presented himself as a self-referrer for oncological screening without subjectively feeling unwell. A large cystic mass lesion can already be seen on the coronal STIR image in the right frontal lobe (left image). The T1-weighted axial and coronal MRI following administration of i.v. Gd-DTPA also shows solid and contrast-enhancing tumor components near the calvaria and at the base of the cyst. The cyst shows an expansive aspect with midline displacement. Histologically the result was shown to be a cystic meningioma.

cally and what the health insurance companies are prepared to finance out of cost-efficiency considerations.

For the time being, it will therefore only be possible to perform whole-body MRI for oncological prevention as part of scientific studies or on the basis of self-referral and in consideration of the existing ambiguities and limitations. Despite the absence of radiation exposure, caution is advised in the unspecific use of whole-body MRI for oncological screening, as neither the effectiveness for the individual nor evidence for larger groups has been verified. Possible risks which result from uncertain diagnoses have been discussed above. On no account should whole-body MRI be promulgated as part of a personal "wellness" program for commercial reasons. Whole-body MRI should also not be understood as a state-supported survey examination.

Certain quality standards for whole-body MRI should indeed be encouraged, and whole-body MRI should be performed in close collaboration with oncological preventative check-ups and consultation, e.g. by primary care physicians/occupational physicians and specialist disciplines such as internists, gynecologists, urologists, etc. Out of a medical sense of responsibility, the customer/patient has to be informed that cancer screening using whole-body MRI is at the beginning of its doubtless promising and certainly rapid development, but is nevertheless not unproblematic at present from several perspectives. The interdisciplinary approach and the demand for quality controls in whole-body MRI oncological screening also necessitate the establishment of networks of competent centers or specialized screening institutions with standardized examination protocols. It would be desirable to combine the results of as many centers or joint scientific data analyses as possible. As long as there is no evidence available from prospective studies for the efficiency of whole-body MRI, the financial responsibility for screening examination beyond scientific studies has to remain with the individual. Whole-body MRI for oncological screening should definitely be considered as a complementary component of cancer prevention carried out in primary medical care, which concentrates on conventional screening measures, such as gynecological examination and mammography, as well as urological examination and the PSA test.

Bibliography

1. Friedenberg RM. The 21st Century: The age of Screening. Radiology 2002; 223: 1–4.
2. Becker N. Screening aus epidemiologischer Sicht. Radiologe 2002; 42: 592–600.
3. Radiation protection enviroment DG – Annual Report 2000. (http://europa.eu.int/comm/environment/radprot/anrep_2000.pdf).
4. Ruehm SG, Goyen M, Barkhausen J, et al. Rapid magnetic resonance angiography for detection of atherosclerosis. Lancet 2001; 357: 1086–91.
5. Gohde S, Goyen M, Forsting M, et al. Prävention ohne Strahlen – eine Strategie zur umfassenden Früherkennung mittels Magnetresonanztomographie (MRT). Radiologe 2002; 42: 622–9.
6. Goehde S, Forsting M, Debatin J. Screening with MRI: A new "all inclusive" Protocol Semin Ultrasound CT MR 2003; 24: 2–11.
7. Goyen M, Goehde SC, Herborn CU, et al. MR-based full-body preventative cardiovascular and tumor imaging: technique and preliminary experiences: Eur Radiol 2004; 14: 783–91.
8. Schlemmer HP, Schäfer J, Pfannenberg C, et al. Fast whole-body assessment of metastatic disease using a novel magnetic resonance imaging system. Invest Radiol 2005; 40(2): 64–71.
9. Gray JAM. Evidence based health care: how to make health policy and management decisions. New York, NY: Churchill Livingstone, 1997.
10. Arbeitsgemeinschaft bevölkerungsbezogener Krebsregister in Deutschland: Krebs in Deutschland. 4. überarbeitete Ausgabe. Saarbrücken, 2004. www.rki.de/KREBS
11. van der Cruijsen-Koeter IW, van der Kwast TH, Schröder FH. Intervall carcinomas in the European Randomized Study of Screening for Prostate Cancer (ERSPC). Rotterdam. J Natl Cancer Inst 2003; 95: 1462–6.
12. Stamey TA, Caldwell M, MyNeal JE, Nolley R, Hemenez M, Downs J. The prostate spezific antigen era in the United States is over for prostate cancer: what happened in the last 20 years? J Urology 2004, 172: 1297–1301.
13. Koans DB, Monsees B, Feig SA. Screening for cancer: when is it valid? – Lessons from the mammography experience. Radiology 2003; 229: 319–27.
14. Humphrey L, Teutsch S, Johnson M. Lung cancer screening with sputum cytologic examination, chest radiography, and computed tomography: An update for the U.S. Preventive services task force. Ann Intern Med 2004; 140: 740–53.

15. Henschke CI, Yankelevitz DF, Kostis WJ. Lungenkrebsscreening? Radiologe 2004; 44: 541–4.

16. Henschke C, Yankelevitz D, Naidich D, et al. CT screening for lung cancer: Suspiciousness of nodules according to size on baseline scans. Radiology 2004; 231: 164–8.

17. Diederich S, Wormanns D, Heindel W. Lungenkrebsfrüherkennung mit Low-dose-CT: ein Update. Radiologe 2002; 42: 608–11.

18. Lutterbey G, Leutner C, Gieseke J, et al. Detektion fokaler Lungenläsionen mit der Magnetresonanz-Tomographie mittels T2-gewichteter Ultrashort-Turbo-Spin-Echo-Sequenz im Vergleich zur Spiral-Computer-Tomographie. Fortschr Röntgenstr 1998; 169: 365–69.

19. Schaefer J, Vollmar J, Schick F, et al. Solitary pulmonary nodules: Dynamic contrast-enhanced MR imaging – perfusion differences in malignant and benign. Radiology 2004; 232(2): 544–53.

20. Ohno Y, Hatabu H, Takenaka D, et al. Solitary pulmonary nodules: Potential role of dynamic MR imaging in management initial experience. Radiology 2002; 224: 503–11.

21. Bond J. Colon polyps and cancer.Endoscopy 2003; 35: 27–35.

22. Smith R, Cokkinides V, Eyre H. American cancer society guidelines for the early detection of cancer, 2004. CA Cancer J Clin 2004; 54: 41–52.

23. Pickhardt P, Choi J, Hwang I, et al. Computed tomographic virtual colonoscopy to screen for colorectal neoplasia in asymptomatic adults. N Engl J Med 2003; 349: 2191–2200.

24. Ajaj W, Pelster G, Treichel U, et al. Dark lumen magnetic resonance colonography: Comparison with conventional colonoscopy for the detection of colorectal pathology. Gut 2003; 52: 1738–43.

25. Schulz K, Kreienberg R, Fischer R, et al. Stufe-3-Leitlinie – Brustkrebs-Früherkennung in Deutschland. Kurzfassung für Ärzte. Radiologe 2003; 43: 495–502.

26. Kneeshaw PJ, Turnbull LW and Drew PJ. Current applications and future direction of MR mammography. Br J Cancer 2003; 88: 4–10.

27. Brown J, Smith RC and Lee CH. Incidental enhancing lesions found on MR imaging of the breast. AJR Am J Roentgenol 2001; 176: 1249–54.

28. Hugosson J, Aus G, Lilja H, et al. Results of a randomized, population-based study of biennial screening using serum prostate-specific antigen measurement to detect prostate carcinoma. Cancer 2004; 100: 1397–1405.

29. Mueller-Lisse U and Mueller-Lisse U. Untersuchungen zur Kosteneffizienz von Screeningmaßnahmen zur Früherkennung des Prostatakarzinoms: Ein Überblick. Radiologe 2002; 42: 601–7.

30. Prostate, Lung, Colorectal and Ovarian Cancer Screening Trial (PLCO) 2004. http://www3.cancer.gov/prevention/plco

31. Mueller-Lisse U, Mueller-Lisse U, Haller S, et al. Likelihood of prostate cancer based on prostate-specific antigen density by MRI : Retrospective analysis. J Comput Assist Tomogr 2002; 26: 432–7.

32. Heuck A, Scheidler J, Sommer B, et al. MR-Tomographie des Prostatakarzinoms. Radiologe 2003; 43: 464–73.

33. Schlemmer H, Merkle J, Grobholz R, et al. Can pre-operative contrast-enhanced dynamic MR imaging for prostate cancer predict microvessel density in prostatectomy specimens? Eur Radiol 2004; 14: 309–17.

34. Togashi K. Ovarian cancer: The clinical role of US, CT, and MRI. Eur Radiol 2003; 13 Suppl 4: L87–104.

35. Fink C, Grenacher L, Hansmann H, et al. Prospektive Studie zum Vergleich der hochauf lösenden Computertomographie und Magnetresonanztomographie in der Detektion von Pankreasneoplasien: Verwendung intravenöser und oraler MR-Kontrastmittel. Fortschr Röntgenstr 2001; 173: 724–30.

36. Düx M, Grenacher L, Lubienski A, et al. Das Magenkarzinom. Stellenwert der bildgebenden Verfahren für Primärdiagnose und präoperatives Tumorstaging. Fortschr Röntgenstr 2000; 172: 661–9.

37. Filipas D, Spix C, Schulz-Lampel D, et al. Sonographisches Screening von Nierenzellkarzinomen. Radiologe 2002; 42: 612–6.

38. Stashuk G. Gastric magnetic resonance study (methods, emiotics). Vestn Rentgenol Radiol 2003; 32–41.

39. Hargaden G, O'Connell M, Kavanagh E, et al. Current concepts in whole-body imaging using turbo short tau inversion recovery MR imaging. AJR 2003; 180: 247–52.

40. Goyen M, Quick HH, Debatin JF, Ladd ME, Barkhausen J, Herborn CU, Bosk S, Kuehl H, Schlepütz M, Ruehm SG. Whole body 3D MR angiography using a rolling table platform: initial clinical experience. Radiology 2002; 224: 270–277.

41. Goyen M, Herborn CU, Kroger K, Lauenstein TC, Debatin JF, Ruehm SG. Detection of atherosclerosis: system imaging for systemic disease with whole-body three-dimensional MR angiography – initial experience. Radiology 2003; 227(1): 277–282.

42. Schäfer JF, Fischmann A, Lichy M, et al. Onkologische Früherkennung mit der Ganzkörper-Magnetresonanztomographie: Möglichkeiten und Grenzen. Radiologe 2004; 44(9): 854–63.

43. Mueller-Horvat C, Radny P, Eigentler TK, et al. Prospective comparison of the impact on treatment decisions of whole-body magnetic resonance imaging and computed tomography in patients with metastatic malignant melanoma. Eur J Cancer 2006; 42: 342–50.

44. Kavanagh E, Smith C and Eustace S. Whole-body turbo stir MR imaging: Controversies and avenues for development. Eur Radiol 2003; 13: 2196–2205.

45. Lauenstein T, Freudenberg L, Goehde S, et al. Whole-body MRI using a rolling table platform for the detection of bone metastases. Eur Radiol 2002; 12: 2091–9.

46. Tausig A, Manthey N, Berger F, et al. Vorzüge und Limitationen der Ganzkörper-Knochenmark-MRT mit Turbo-STIR-Sequenzen im Vergleich zur planaren Skelettszintigraphie. Nuklearmedizin 2000; 39: 174–9.

47. Walker R, Kessar P, Blanchard R, et al. Turbo stir magnetic resonance imaging as a whole body screening tool for metastases in patients with breast carcinoma: Preliminary clinical experience. J Magn Reson Imaging 2000; 11: 343–50.

Susanne C. Ladd

12.1 Screening: Definitions and requirements

Entering the term "screening" in databases such as Medline, one obtains almost 200,000 hits. On closer examination, however, it becomes apparent that "screening" is usually used in a rather "loose" sense, such as for the search for tumors in an individual ("we screen the patient for tumors"). This does not do justice to the epidemiological sense of the word and can lead to interpretation problems in research results. For this reason, the term "screening" will firstly be defined, and the requirements for effective and successful screening, primarily in radiology, will be described.

12.1.1 Types of prevention

Prevention "of/against diseases" describes general attempts to reduce morbidity and mortality in the population group studied and to do so under justifiable "conditions". In this context, "primary prevention" is understood as the reduction of risk factors to avoid the occurrence of certain diseases. The impact of primary prevention has been known for more than 2000 years; the physician and philosopher Maimonides (1135–1204) once said: "Live sensibly – among a thousand people only one dies a natural death; the rest succumb to irrational modes of living".

Examples of primary prevention include adding fluoride to drinking water and mandatory seat belt usage in cars. In the medical world, vaccination reduces the occurrence of infectious diseases, and the control of cardiovascular risk factors, such as arterial hypertension, obesity, smoking, or hyperlipidemia, is known to reduce the occurrence of cardiovascular events.

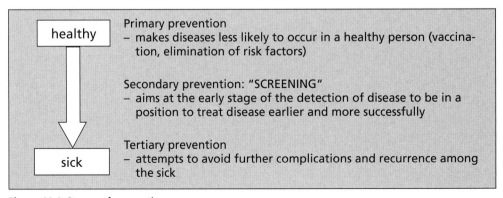

Figure 11.1 Stages of prevention.

Secondary prevention describes the search for – still – occult or non-symptomatic diseases. For instance, the glucose tolerance test serves to identify diabetes mellitus at an early stage. The success of secondary preventive measures of course depends on the availability of an effective therapy for the target disease.

But how should the asymptomatic "screening participant" be called? He/she is not yet a "patient", but perhaps a "volunteer" in the context of studies. A single individual who undergoes screening could, for example, be termed a "client". The term "volunteer" will be used in this chapter in the context of secondary prevention.

Tertiary prevention serves to avoid deterioration in condition given the presence of a known disease. Beta-receptor blockers to reduce mortality in patients following myocardial infarct or regular ophthalmological check-ups for early diagnosis of a retinopathy among diabetics are examples of tertiary prevention (Fig. 12.1).

12.1.2   What does "screening" mean?

The term "screening" is normally used for secondary prevention measures: Screening describes a routine examination of a defined group of persons to identify diseases or risk factors at an early stage. That is why screening is often termed "preventive medical examination or checkup". The term screening will be used in this sense in the following. The aim of a screening program in the medical field is to increase the life expectancy of the examinees with life threatening diseases and to enhance quality of life. The most accurate examination methods possible should be used to identify as many diseases as possible still in their non-symptomatic phase, so that early treatment or change in life style can be initiated.

The requirements for effective screening are summarized in Figure 12.2, but will be explained in detail as follows.

1. Disease: How impaired is the population through the disease with regard to its possible consequences:
   - death
   - course of the disease
   - disability
   - costs for the general public without early diagnosis
   - pain
   - well-being
   - poverty

   Screening methods: How good is the screening test in relation to
   - sensitivity
   - specificity
   - simplicity
   - availability
   - costs
   - safety
   - acceptance

   Therapy options: How effective are the therapy options in relation to
   - difference in effectiveness between early and delayed therapy
   - patient compliance

Figure 12.2 Criteria for the inclusion of a disease in a screening program.

12.1.3   Requirements for the target disease

12.1.3.1 Prevalence

One of the essential requirements for cost-effective screening is a sufficiently high prevalence of the target disease in the population group examined. Dependent on the costs for the screening test, the prevalence should be at least 5–10%. The inherent low prevalence of most diseases, at least in the general population, leads to a very low positive predictive value for many screening tests irrespective of the disease investigated, even if the accuracy of the test is very high (Bayes' Theorem). This would indicate that a large number of examinations on ultimately healthy persons have to be performed in order to discover just a few cases of disease. The prevalence of a disease can be elevated in a group of individuals for which risk factors are known; these make the disease more probable, e.g. considering the risk factor "age" for breast carcinoma or colorectal carcinoma as a preselection criterium.

12.1.3.2 Anticipated success of treatment

Apart from an adequate prevalence of the disease screened for, the following requirement for effective screening should also be fulfilled: the target disease should, if it remains untreated, be accompanied with a high morbidity and mortality, and treatment at an early stage should show a significantly improved outcome. Otherwise the screening would not lead to an improvement in quality of life and would therefore be senseless; the volunteer would be unnecessarily burdened by their possibly unfavorable diagnosis.

Diseases that are reasonable to screen for include colon carcinoma, breast carcinoma, bronchial carcinoma, and atherosclerosis in its many manifestations. This is due to the good treatment options available for the early stages of the disease, but also to the high prevalence in the general population.

12.1.4   Requirements for a screening test

12.1.4.1 Availability

The ideal screening test should be available ubiquitously, such that all persons falling into a screening category can be examined. This raises the benefit of screening; at the same time, a "fair" distribution of screening examinations can take place.

12.1.4.2 Costs

The screening test should only require a low level of resources for its realization and interpretation. Furthermore, it must be considered that the costs also include any additional indirect examinations, which are for example required in the case of unclear results.

12.1.4.3 Diagnostic accuracy

High accuracy and conclusiveness for a screening test, as described by the parameters of sensitivity, specificity, positive and negative predictive values, may reduce the number of additional examinations required in the case of unclear results, thereby considerably reducing the follow-on costs.

12.1.4.4 Tolerance

Another important aspect the screening test has to fulfill is that it shows no (or a low, acceptable degree of) side effects. While it is ethically justified to accept certain risks in a diagnostic technique for patients with disease symptoms or known diseases, for the usually healthy individual undergoing a screening program this only applies to a very limited degree.

12.1.4.5 Acceptance in the population

The major significance the acceptance of a test has on the success of screening measures can be illustrated with the example of cervical carcinoma. Women with the highest risk of developing cervical carcinoma very seldom go for a preventive examination, and the disease is therefore often only diagnosed at an advanced stage. Only if a large proportion of persons for whom a screening measure is foreseen also take part in the screening program can the target disease be reduced in the general population.

However, the acceptance among physicians also plays a role: Screening tests are sometimes not performed because the physician considers them too time-consuming or laborious; this category of examinations sometimes also includes colonoscopy. The simplification of screening tests must continue to be perused to improve acceptance from all involved; information should be disseminated to a greater extent than has previously been the case, so that the physician as well as the volunteer can be more convinced to accept the effort entailed with an examination.

12.1.5   What can screening lead to?

12.1.5.1 Consequences of successful screening

Screening tests more often yield true-negative results than true-positive results, as the prevalence of the disease intended to be detected lies usually below 50%. If a screening test yields a true-negative result, the examination is concluded.

In the case of true-positive results, either the appropriate therapy is immediately initiated, which can include risk factor reduction or chemotherapy or an operation or further examinations which have to be carried out to specify the stage of the disease or its consequences more precisely. Unfortunately, after his/her assessment of the images, the radiologist does not know whether the diagnosis is correct or whether a false result has been obtained.

12.1.5.2 Consequences of incorrect results

The accuracy of medical tests, including radiological techniques, never reaches 100%. This means that erroneous or uncertain results can always arise. False-negative results do not have any immediate consequences for the radiologist or volunteer, but ultimately the op-

portunity for early therapy of the non-detected disease is missed, with the related reper-
cussions for the volunteer, but also theoretically for the radiologist (lawsuits).

False-positive results lead to additional diagnostic measures, assuming the volunteer
does not refuse. There may also be invasive examinations, such as biopsy or open surgery
of an uncertain lung lesion. This not only leads to increased overall costs, but possibly also
to deterioration in the state of health of the volunteer, who is retrospectively seen to have
been "healthy" prior to the screening test. The consequences not only have physical implications, but also affect the psyche.

12.1.5.3 Psychological implications: "Labeling" of the patient

Negative labeling: Results of medical examinations can have a severe impact on the psyche
of the volunteer. A positive test result can result in negative psychologic effects ("negative
labeling"): the volunteer can for instance develop a carcinophobia, which also remains after healing and deters them from visiting physicians in the future. This is especially common in the case of breast carcinoma patients [1]. At this point it is insignificant whether the
test led to a true-positive or a false-positive result. Negative labeling is especially problematic from an ethical viewpoint, because it can lead to a continuous feeling of fear and threat
rather than an improved state of health.

Positive labeling: However, the opposite, "positive labeling", can arise for a true-negative or a false-negative test result: The volunteer is pleased about his/her confirmed good
health and has the feeling that he/she will stay fit for work for many years to come just as
they have always been. But also in this case, a negative effect is conceivable if the volunteer,
for example, avoids going to the physician for many years to come and so forgoes the op-
portunity of early diagnosis of diseases in the future.

12.1.5.4 Definition of "health"

This aspect, often not considered by the physician, is addressed by the World Health Or-
ganization in its current definition of "health": "Health" is a state of complete physical,
mental, and social well-being and is therefore not merely the absence of disease or infir-
mity. It will become increasingly necessary in the future to also consider the psychological
component of health, as indicated here.

12.2 Screening in radiology

12.2.1 History

Radiology classically investigates the symptomatic, individual patient; the term "screening" is often used in this context to describe the search for diseases in the individual. If the
term "prevention" is applied to the classical functions of radiology, this usually relates to
tertiary prevention. Screening in the sense of early diagnosis of diseases has until now been
primarily the domain of the clinical specialties that work with physical examinations or
blood tests, for example.

Possibly the first actual screening program based on radiological imaging and, at the
same time, one of the first screening programs per se, was the widespread X-ray imaging

of the lung in the 1950s. It only served to benefit the well-being of the individual in a secondary sense; it was primarily designed to identify potentially infectious individuals with tuberculosis, to treat them, and therefore to eliminate the sources of infection for the general population. Effective primary prevention was thus carried out for the general population. Two developments formed the condition for effective screening here: firstly, the introduction of a mobile, miniature X-ray system in the 1930s by Russell Reynolds and Watsons Ltd [2] (high availability, controllable costs, sufficient accuracy, limited side effects), and secondly, the development of effective antibiotic therapy techniques in the 1950s.

Breast screening was introduced for the first time two decades later. Breast screening is a classical example of secondary prevention: The aim is the earliest possible identification and, consequently, early therapy of malignant breast lesions and therefore a reduction in morbidity and mortality in the group of women affected. Whereas breast screening is already established in the USA and some European countries [3, 4], in Germany a heated debate continues on the benefits and risks of general screening in the unselected population [5].

12.2.2 The latest developments in radiology

Multi-slice computed tomography (CT) has been investigated in recent years as a screening technique. As a result of its high diagnostic accuracy and short examination time, this technique is well suited for the detection of many diseases. Studies have particularly focused on cardiovascular diseases [6], bronchial carcinoma [7, 8], and colon carcinoma [9].

In recent times, whole-body examinations can be carried out using CT systems with an especially large number of detector rings without compromising spatial resolution. These whole-body CT screening examinations are primarily offered in the USA [10].

12.2.3 Problems with ionizing radiation

All these examinations are accompanied by often significant radiation exposure. The associated risks have led the Federal Drug Administration (FDA) to issue radiation alerts [11, 12]. Nevertheless, the number of centers offering CT screening continues to rise, at least in the USA [13].

The European Union has banned screening techniques that are accompanied by ionizing radiation. To date, no radiological screening examinations are allowed by law in Germany [14]; the only exception was passed by the Federal Standing Committee of Physicians and Health Insurers at the end of 2003 for mammography screening [15] after several studies had revealed a positive balance between benefit and risk [16]. According to EU guidelines, mammography screening can only be carried out under stringent quality assurance conditions [17, 18]. Here screening means sacrificing the requirement for a justified indication in the individual case if this coincides with a benefit for the group of persons examined. "According to the German X-ray Ordinance, widespread X-ray survey examinations for breast cancer screening represent an application outside of medical science in the strict sense, as they do not pertain to a patient with a result requiring clarification. Examinations of this type must be specially approved in accordance with Article 25, Paragraph 1, Clause 2 of the German X-ray Ordinance (RöV) to ensure that radiation protection is appropriately observed. The legal approval overrules the requirement for a justified indication otherwise required in the individual case, which stipulates that the health benefits of the procedure outweigh the associated radiation risk. The bodies responsible for issuing such approvals are the highest health authorities in the federal states of Germany, which implement the X-ray Ordinance on behalf of the federal government. Without this approval, mammography screening is not allowed to commence" [19].

Apart from the exceptions stated above, this implies that all (!) radiological examinations with ionizing radiation must be individually indicated, as is also the case in clinical routine. Usually, this will not apply to screening examinations.

For this reason the focus of European interest is placed on an imaging technique that does not involve X-rays and hazardous side effects: magnetic resonance imaging (MRI) [20].

12.2.4   Why screening with MRI?

MRI is the imaging technique of choice in clinical routine work for assessing a wide range of diseases. Nearly all organ systems can be very precisely investigated with MRI; from a purely technical perspective, MRI can therefore be used as a screening test for all these technically presentable diseases.

Compared with computed tomography, which is accompanied by radiation exposure, the risks of an MRI examination are minimal; no detrimental side effects have occurred to date in clinically approved examinations [20]. However, intravenous contrast agents, which are often an integral component of the examination, are associated with undesirable effects in individual cases. Even though these are rare, an anaphylactic reaction can indeed occur. Compared with contrast agents containing iodine, the paramagnetic MRI contrast agents approved so far are not nephrotoxic in the normal dosages [21, 22, 23]. On account of this low side-effect profile, MRI is increasingly accepted as a radiological examination modality not only by physicians, but also in the general population; in particular, an MRI examination is already in demand as a "screening technique" among health-conscious persons who can afford this examination themselves. This self-referral type of examination does not comply with the definition of screening, however, as there is no precise definition or characterization of the group of examinees.

Single organ screening for the most important diseases will be briefly introduced here, because the evidence regarding indications, possibilities, and limitations is partly transferable to whole-body screening as it is possible today. The advantages and disadvantages of whole-body MR examinations will then be presented.

12.3   Single organ screening

Until now, the restricted field of view of MR systems generally only allowed the examination of single organs. These cannot usually be combined in a single session for logistical reasons (multiple dynamic sequences following application of contrast agent) or for reasons of time (acceptance of the overall examination time). The first screening studies in radiology were therefore limited to single organs.

12.3.1 Tumors

The term "screening" is used in oncology to describe the search for metastases in patients with known primary tumors. The cost-effectiveness of metastasis screening is not known precisely for all types of tumors; as the sub-group of tumor patients is relatively small, consensus prevails as to the necessity and the moral obligation to thoroughly examine these patients, because the therapy can vary from surgery to adjunctive or palliative therapy depending on the stage of the disease. Tumor screening is also suitable, at least technically, for secondary prevention as demonstrated by the following examples.

12.3.1.1 Bronchial carcinoma

Current bronchial carcinoma screening measures reflect the significantly higher chances of therapy success at the earliest possible stage. Due to its inherently high spatial image resolution, computed tomography (CT) represents the method of choice for the detection of malignant lung lesions, also in their early stages. The radiation exposure associated with CT has, however, so far restricted its use as a screening method even among the risk populations.

MRI of the lung was, until recently, unsuitable for the detection of small pulmonary lesions due to the susceptibility effects on the margins between the interstitium and the air-filled alveoli. Turbo spin-echo sequences with ultra-short echo times often completely suppress these artifacts and lead to a promisingly high sensitivity in the detection of lesions above 10 mm in size [24, 25]. Small, partly calcified lesions are not detected due to the lack of signal-enhancing spins, and very small lesions under 3 mm are only rarely detectable. Research has to reveal whether these advancements may even lead to an increase in specificity and hence to a partial advantage over CT, which is not very specific.

12.3.1.2 Prostate carcinoma

Prostate carcinomas are today diagnosed on the basis of various examinations (measurement of prostate-specific antigen, palpation, and, if necessary, transrectal ultrasound and biopsies). In comparison, MRI has demonstrated its potential for precise localization and staging of a carcinoma in clinical studies [26, 27].

Unpleasant endorectal coils are often no longer used today; suitable combinations of new surface coils are usually sufficient to achieve adequate image resolution, and this raises patient acceptance significantly. However, larger prospective studies on the use of MRI as a screening method are still outstanding.

12.3.1.3 Breast carcinoma

The dependence of the prognosis on the time of detection (tumor stage) for breast carcinoma is well-known [28] and has led many countries to offer conventional mammography as a screening measure starting at a certain age; however, this is accompanied by low accuracy and very high radiation exposure.

MR mammography, on the other hand, is a significantly more accurate method of detecting breast carcinoma [29], although the challenge of raising the hitherto inadequate specificity will continue in the years to come. MR mammography is currently used especially as a screening technique to detect secondary tumors prior to planned operations or for precise characterization of unclear mammography results. MRI is especially effective in identifying genetically linked breast carcinoma, which, on account of the high gland density of the generally young patients, often cannot be identified using conventional mammography [30]; at the same time, radiation exposure of these patients is to be avoided in view of the higher radiation sensitivity of the mammary gland tissue. Sensitivity and specificity of MRI for this purpose are 100% and 95% [31]. Also in the case of breast carcinoma, the effectiveness of MRI largely depends on the sufficiently high prevalence of the disease in the group of women examined, which can be obtained by effective preselection of the volunteers.

12.3.1.4 Colon carcinoma

Colorectal carcinoma is an especially well-suited example of a disease whose early diagnosis leads to an improved prognosis: The prevalence of colorectal carcinoma is very high, even in the unselected general population. Approximately 6% of the general population will develop a colorectal carcinoma in the course of their lives [32]. The disease is lethal if it is diagnosed too late and has significantly better chances for healing if diagnosed in its early stage. The special biology of the colorectal carcinoma, which usually develops over a long period of time from a precancerous polyp to a fully formed carcinoma [33], has made colonoscopy a promising screening method in medicine, at least in theory [34]. However, the acceptance of this screening method within the population due to the necessary laxative measures and partly the pain associated with colonoscopy is limited. This reduces the effect of today's screening measures; despite worldwide campaigns, incidence of the disease continues to rise [35]. Alternative screening techniques, which are better accepted by the general population, are urgently needed to control this common disease.

The introduction of CT and MR colonography was encouraging in this regard [36]. Polyps above a size of 8 mm are identified very reliably [37, 38, 39]; this is quite adequate for effective screening in light of the growth properties of colonic carcinoma [40]. The preparation time (colon cleansing on the evening before the examination) and the actual examination time are considerably shorter than for conventional colonoscopy, and the examinations are objectively far more tolerable and can therefore be performed without pain medication or sedatives.

Several sequences are available to assess the colon, which is distended after administration of a spasmolyticum by an enema using air or aqueous solution. They differ in the signal from the enema and the colon wall. Today, a gradient-echo sequence with T2/T1 contrast as a "bright lumen" technique or a T1-weighted gradient-echo sequence before and after intravenous administration of contrast agent is usually used. The latter is particularly suitable for differentiating any stool residues (these are hyperintense already in pre-contrast images) from colon wall lesions (these only yield a signal after administration of contrast agent [41]).

Extremely promising efforts are currently aimed towards making colon cleansing superfluous. Oral contrast agents are used to adapt the signal of the stool to that of the enema, so that one can "see through the stool" [42]; confusion with colon wall lesions should thus ideally be excluded.

A special advantage of MRI, however, lies in the extended field of view: Beyond the mucous tissue of the colon, it should be possible to assess the outer colon layers and furthermore also the organs of the upper abdomen; thus, evidence can be found simultaneously on the presence e.g. of hepatic metastases.

The costs for MR colonoscopy usually lie in the same region as those for colonoscopy [37], so that at least a certain prospect of cost acceptance by the health insurance companies exists once the promising results so far are also confirmed in the long term.

12.3.2 Atherosclerosis

Most clinical or radiological diagnostic techniques for vascular pathologies are either imprecise in localizing and ascertaining severity or are restricted to a limited field of view, which is inadequate for the systemic nature of the disease. Computed tomography, although it does in principle produce high-resolution images [43], also has to be included in this group, since in such cases it requires such a high radiation dosage that it can hardly be used as a "whole-body" screening examination. The invasive, more expensive examinations and those involving radiation exposure are restricted to individual volunteers who are symptomatic or at least show a high "pretest probability" of arterial pathologies.

12.3.2.1 Peripheral atherosclerosis

MR angiography produces good results comparable with conventional angiography in almost all arterial vascular regions, including the carotid arteries [44], the renal arteries [45], and the peripheral vessels [46, 47, 48, 49]. Today arteries can be examined from "head to foot" with a single application of contrast agent; the results are three dimensional, high quality, easy to post-process, and accurate angiograms [50, 51], which, at least in the larger radiological centers, have largely replaced diagnostic catheter angiographies for the assessment of these vessels.

Due to the high prevalence of atherosclerosis in the population, the large number of known risk factors, which allow effective preselection of those volunteers likely to be affected by atherosclerosis, and the high level of therapy success once the disease is identified at an early stage, screening measures are generally effective. MR angiography is a technique available to the physician and volunteer which, within minutes, can reveal vessels not yet significantly affected in the asymptomatic individual. The comparison of costs between the conventional procedure (several days hospitalization, multiple not very accurate or invasive examinations, possible limitation to one or a few territories) and this new approach (outpatient MR angiography) is of course not easy to carry out; however, hard data in this regard would be of enormous importance for future discussions with the referrers.

12.3.2.2 Coronary heart disease

Coronary heart disease (CHD) is one of the leading causes of death in the western world [52]. Whereas the known risk factors can be ascertained by physical examination, laboratory tests, and medical history, MRI offers the possibility of identifying damage to the heart muscle that has already occurred. The direct depictability of at least the proximal coronary segments and perfusion examinations of the myocardium also provide evidence of early stages of disease. It is also the case for coronary heart disease that the prospects of success are significantly raised by early intervention, whether through reduction in risk factors, medication, or minimally invasive therapies.

As in the examination of peripheral vessels, until now rather inaccurate or more invasive diagnostic methods have been available for the detection of CHD. Cardiac MRI today allows non-invasive examination of regional and global contractility [53, 54], heart valve function and morphology [55], myocardial perfusion, and myocardial viability [56, 57, 58]. Although MRI is competitive or even more accurate than competing techniques [59] in many fields of investigation, MRI still suffers from its too low spatial resolution in the direct presentation of the distal segments of the coronaries, which still limits its sensitivity for coronary stenoses. The examination of myocardial perfusion under stress conditions (induced in MRI mainly by medication) can compensate for the absence of direct coronary imaging, as the perfusion of affected coronaries differs from the normal coronaries even in a very early stage of stenosis [60]. However, stress perfusion is a complex and not completely hazard-free technique. The screening examination for CHD therefore remains limited primarily to movement disorders, myocardial infarcts, and possibly to the direct imaging of the proximal coronary arteries.

12.3.2.3 Cerebrovascular diseases

The head is the region of the body that was most often examined at the beginning of MRI development and still is today. Inflammatory, neoplastic, degenerative, and vascular diseases can be assessed very reliably [61, 62]. The established spin-echo-based sequences for the presentation of morphology have been supplemented in recent years by complex techniques which reflect the functional processes in the brain ("blood oxygen level dependent imaging", "diffusion weighted imaging", etc.).

Atherosclerosis screening must allow both extracranial as well as intracranial arterial vessels to be imaged with high spatial resolution. This is still one of the few remaining indications for time-of-flight sequences in many clinical departments. The small intracerebral vessels can be thus imaged in patients who have already suffered a cerebrovascular event; previously asymptomatic individuals, especially those from risk groups, can also be examined easily and quickly. The size, number, and distribution pattern of ischemic regions usually allow the possible etiologies to be derived; microangiopathic damage of the white substance indicates a prolonged arterial hypertony [63], whereas thromboembolic changes can usually be explained by severe carotid stenoses. MRI is certainly in a position to quantify vessel wall changes as the most important prognostic criterium for cerebral insults and to partly characterize vessel wall components; until now, however, this has required the procurement of high-resolution surface coils and the use of several different MR sequences. The investment in time for volunteers, as well as medical-technical personnel, is certainly still too high for use as a screening examination. Ultrasound-based examination techniques are better suited for this application, but they cannot image the complete anatomy of the vessels as MRI can, especially the components near the base of the skull.

12.3.3 Arrhythmogenic right ventricular dysplasia

The suspicion of an arrhythmogenic right ventricular dysplasia (ARVD) usually exists after an event triggered by a ventricular tachycardia. As ARVD includes a genetic component, non-symptomatic family members of someone affected are often screened for this disease. MRI, with its high soft tissue contrast, allows not only a high degree of detection and localization of fatty components in the myocardium, but also the assessment of right ventricular form and function. Right ventricular signs of ARVD in MRI correlate well with evoked potentials, which has resulted in MRI being increasingly used as a screening measure [64, 65].

12.3.4   MR venography

Pulmonary angiographies have been performed with MRI for a long time now in many clinical departments as a single-station examination. They can be easily combined with the examination of veins of the lower extremities and the pelvis to verify thromboembolic origin, also in patients with paradoxical embolisms [66]. Another typical indication for whole-body MRI is clarification of the extent and localization of arteriovenous malformations.

12.3.5   Whole-body measurement of muscle and fat mass

The possibility of imaging the whole body in axial slices with MRI also opens up the possibility of determining the total fat content or the muscle mass of a person [67, 68] (also see Chap. 10). The latter can, for example, be used to measure the effectiveness of training [69]. It is also known that the fat distribution (subcutaneous versus intraabdominal fat) is of prognostic importance for cardiovascular events [70]. Whole-body MRI also shows itself to be useful in the case of other systemic diseases, either to determine the propagation of a disease [71, 72], such as polymyositis or muscular dystrophies [73], or to measure therapy success.

12.3.6   Fetal malformations

The use of MRI as a screening technique for fetuses has shifted to the center of attention at the moment. Here, imaging is particularly reliant on fast sequences with little susceptibility to motion artifacts. Especially successful are T2-weighted fast turbo-spin sequences with a high turbo factor in various planes angled to the structures of interest. The focus of attention is on the early and, above all, accurate diagnosis and characterization of cerebrospinal malformations. Another interesting indication is presented in the determination of fetal cerebral oxygenation in risk groups (placental insufficiency) [74].

Even sequences with high incident radio frequency energy do not lead to a significant increase in temperature in the region of the fetus [75]. Animal experiments on embryonic or blastocyte development after exposure to MRI or MR contrast agents have, however, been contradictory in the past [76, 77, 78]. Thus, there is a wide consensus that female patients in the first trimester should only be examined with MRI after a careful assessment of the indication, also for psychological reasons: If there is a detrimental development, the suspicion of damage through the MRI cannot usually be refuted.

12.4 Whole-body MR screening

The possibility of not only examining limited regions of the body, but also the whole body in its entirety, with one or more sequences has attracted special interest in recent times. This necessitated a series of developments to facilitate more robust, faster, and spatially higher resolving image acquisition.

12.4.1 Technical requirements

The rapid advancements in MRI systems, with their remarkable reduction in image acquisition time combined with newly developed moving table techniques, allow the coverage of more than one body region or organ system (also see Chap. 1). Suitable combinations of MR sequences can therefore, in theory, be used for cost-effective screening. The acceleration in image acquisition can be utilized to reduce the examination time for the volunteer, or more images can be acquired in the same time, such that the application spectra of MRI and CT merge to some extent. At the same time, the advantages of MRI over CT of inherent high soft tissue contrast, the arbitrary choice of slice orientation, and the option of three-dimensional imaging remain. These useful characteristics mean that pathomorphological changes can be identified with greater certainty and at an earlier stage with MRI.

12.4.2 Applications

There are nevertheless only few studies in the current literature which use MRI as a controlled screening examination; there are hardly any studies that extend beyond single organ screening, as used for breast and colon carcinomas, to whole-body examination strategies.

There are essentially two groups of patients for whom "real" whole-body MR screening protocols have been applied on a somewhat larger scale so far. These firstly include tumor patients, which has been described previously (see also Chap. 6, 7, 8, and 11). This falls under the category "tertiary prevention".

Secondly, risk patients for vascular disease are at the focus of interest, primarily because atherosclerosis is the number one cause of death. The patients are predominantly preselected, in that arteriosclerotic changes have been identified in one or more other territories or they fulfill a particular risk profile, which increases the prevalence for the region examined. The individual vessel stenoses do not need to have led to symptoms, though.

However, the new "revolutionary" idea for radiology has been to apply such whole-body protocols on non-symptomatic volunteers as part of a secondary screening program.

12.4.3 Combined atherosclerosis and tumor protocol

A protocol for a comprehensive examination, not only of the vascular system, is presented as follows (Table 12.1). Due to the systemic nature of atherosclerosis, a specific screening protocol has to demonstrate high accuracy in the detection of vascular changes over several regions of the body. This includes the cerebrovascular system with its extracerebral and intra-

Table 12.1 Protocol for a whole-body MRI examination for atherosclerosis and colonic polyps. The total examination time ("in-room time") is approx. 60 min. SE: spin-echo sequence; TSE: turbo spin-echo sequence; CA: contrast agent; FLAIR: fluid-attenuated inversion recovery sequence; HASTE: half-Fourier single-shot turbo spin-echo sequence; trueFISP: true fast imaging with steady-state precession

Examination	Sequence	Special features
MRI of the head	T1w SE axial	Unenhanced
	T2w TSE axial	
	2D inversion recovery FLAIR axial	
	Diffusion-weighted echo planar imaging axial	
Whole-body MR angiography	3D spoiled gradient-echo sequence coronal	Individual bolus timing in the ascending aorta; double dose CA diluted to 60 ml; injection protocol: 30 ml at 1.2 ml/s, 30 ml at 0.7 ml/s, and NaCl flush at 1.2 ml/s
MRI of the heart	2D HASTE axial	Covers heart and entire lung
	2D trueFISP short axis ("shared phases"), as well as two, three, and four chamber view	Detects motion disorders and valve pathologies
	2D inversion recovery gradient-echo sequence ("late enhancement") long axis	Uses CA administration from MR angiography; no repeated administration of CA
	3D inversion recovery gradient-echo sequence ("late enhancement") short axis	
MR colonography	3D spoiled gradient-echo sequence coronal	Prior to and 75 seconds after single dose of CA at 2 ml/s
MRI of the head	Contrast-enhanced T1w gradient-echo sequence axial	Uses the CA previously applied

cerebral arteries, as well as the parenchyma supplied by these vessels. It is really rather difficult to predict cerebrovascular disease; only 26–50% of patients with a peripheral vascular occlusive disease (PVOD) have a cerebral component [79, 80]; many patients with a vascular disease are however only diagnosed once they have become symptomatic [81].

The screening protocol for atherosclerosis also includes the vascular examination of the aorta, supraaortal branches, visceral vessels, and the periphery. The possibility of imaging all these vessels in a single, brief examination has significantly changed the diagnostic procedure in centers having his facility. Finally, the heart should be examined (Fig. 12.3, 12.4). Even though the examination may often "only" be able to look for wall motion disorders and previous cardiac infarcts for reasons of time pressure or the lack of suitable sequences, even this provides important information, since the rate of unknown cardiac infarcts/unidentified CHD is not inconsiderable [82].

A sufficiently comprehensive combination protocol for the radiological screening of two particularly common and potentially lethal diseases – atherosclerosis and colon carcinoma – is described in [83]. The protocol optimizes the logistics of contrast agent administration, which is not trivial if several individual examinations are to be performed in a single session without impairment of quality; it offers the examination quality commonly found in clinical routine and can be performed within 60 min (Table 12.1).

The head is examined according to clinical standards. This includes diffusion-weighted sequences and 3D time-of-flight (TOF) MR angiography. After completion of all other subsequent examination components, for which contrast agent has been applied in the meantime, a T1-weighted sequence of the head is acquired, which increases the sensitivity for the detection of potential cerebral tumors.

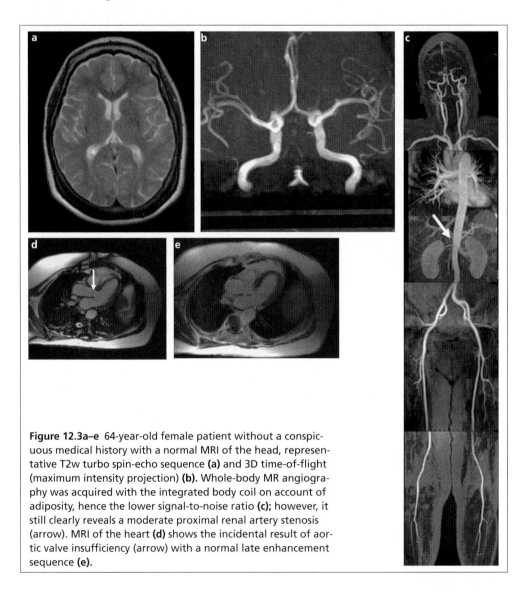

Figure 12.3a–e 64-year-old female patient without a conspicuous medical history with a normal MRI of the head, representative T2w turbo spin-echo sequence **(a)** and 3D time-of-flight (maximum intensity projection) **(b)**. Whole-body MR angiography was acquired with the integrated body coil on account of adiposity, hence the lower signal-to-noise ratio **(c)**; however, it still clearly reveals a moderate proximal renal artery stenosis (arrow). MRI of the heart **(d)** shows the incidental result of aortic valve insufficiency (arrow) with a normal late enhancement sequence **(e)**.

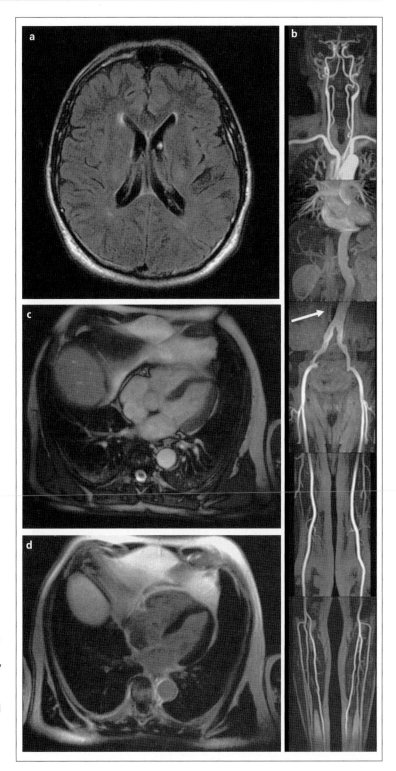

Figure 12.4a–d
64-year-old volunteer without a conspicuous medical history with mild cerebral microangiopathy **(a)**, a previously unidentified abdominal aortic aneurysm of 5 cm with thrombus margin (arrow) and ectactic pelvic arteries as revealed by whole-body MR angiography **(b)** (image with the Angio*SURF* system and surface coils), and normal MRI of the heart function **(c)** and the myocardium **(d)**.

The whole-body MR angiography was performed with the aid of a system-compatible "roller-mounted table platform" (back then the newer systems with integrated whole-body image acquisition were not yet available) [50]. This platform allows acquisition of 5–6 three-dimensional angiography data sets following a single administration of contrast agent using the "bolus chase" technique. Besides the possibility of now covering a field of view in excess of 180 cm without repositioning the volunteer, an advantage of this system is the use of surface coils, which, thanks to their higher signal-to-noise ratio, deliver significantly improved image quality compared to the body coil integrated into the scanner.

Heart imaging involves an axial T2-weighted "dark-blood" sequence to produce a morphological overview; this is however extended in the craniocaudal direction to include the entire lung. Images of this type are very sensitive for the detection of focal lung nodules [84]. Functional imaging with fast gradient-echo sequences (T2/T1 contrasts are most informative), as well as late enhancement sequences using inversion recovery sequences to optimize the contrast of infarctions versus healthy myocardium, are acquired in several short and long axis sections. Here, late enhancement imaging uses the intravenous contrast agent previously applied for MR angiography, and repeated administration of contrast agent is not required.

In the last part of the whole-body MRI, attention is then turned to malignomas, and MR colonography is performed (Fig. 12.5). Colon carcinoma, as the second most frequent malignant cause of death after bronchial carcinoma, is the special focus of attention. A three-dimensional T1-weighted gradient-echo sequence is acquired following spasmolysis and rectal enema [85].

In unselected volunteers, who were above all characterized by the fact that they were interested in such screening measures (average age 51 years), the rate of significant atherosclerotic findings was rather low [83, 86] (myocardial infarcts 0.3%, strokes 0.6%, significant carotid stenosis 1%, significant renal artery stenoses 0.3%, significant peripheral stenoses 1%); colonic polyps were diagnosed in 4% of cases, there were no colonic carcinomas. Of course, the prevalence of such conditions also depends on age. It is, however, as yet unknown whether the persons with positive results take the diagnosed disease seriously and take advantage of therapeutic measures, such as risk factor reduction or the regulation of hypertension with drugs.

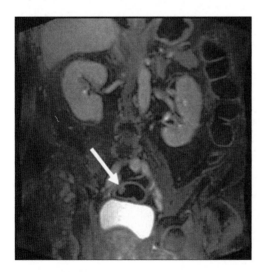

Figure 12.5 57-year-old volunteer with a small polyp in the sigmoid colon. T1w 3D gradient-echo sequence using the "dark lumen" technique after administration of intravenous contrast agent.

12.4.4 Secondary results

Of special interest, but also especially unclear, is what the radiologist should do with the more frequent "secondary results" or incidental findings. He/she cannot only concentrate on the target disease (atherosclerotic changes in vessels, heart, and head, or colon lesions); especially three-dimensional imaging and repeated coverage of the abdomen in the arterial phase (MR angiography) and the portal-venous and venous phases (MR colonography) are known to yield particularly accurate information on pathologies in other organs and structures [87], starting with the parenchymal organs of the upper abdomen and extending across all bone and soft tissue structures in the field of view through to lymph nodes and the venous system. The pathologies that can be discovered include very rare malignomas (Fig. 12.6); renal cell carcinomas or suspected lung lesions are the most common, although they only occurred in [86] in just 0.6% of cases. Even benign results can impair quality of life, such as axial hiatal hernias of the stomach, cerebral aneurysms, heart valve defects, prostate hypertrophy, herniated vertebral discs, and others.

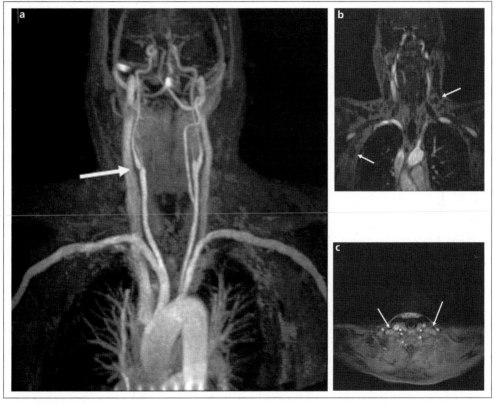

Figure 12.6a–c 63-year-old volunteer with Hodgkin's disease diagnosed 3 years ago; he came for atherosclerosis screening. The first station of MR angiography shows a previously unknown circular constriction of the right internal carotid artery (arrow) in the maximum intensity projection **(a)**; the source images **(b)** lead to the suspicion of cervical, supraclavicular, and axillary lymph node infiltration, which was confirmed in the delayed contrast images not only here **(c)**, but also in the abdomen and pelvis. The volunteer was hospitalized for renewed therapy of the lymphoma.

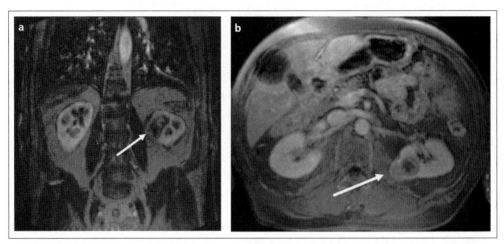

Figure 12.7a, b Secondary result in a whole-body MRI for a 63-year-old volunteer without symptoms. The coronal source image from the second station of the contrast-enhanced 3D MR angiography **(a)** shows a lesion in the left kidney, which can be diagnosed with certainty as a renal cell carcinoma with the subsequent axial 3D gradient-echo sequence **(b)** (arrow).

Non-vascular pathologies are often just "surmised" and cannot be characterized in more detail (Fig. 12.7). It is certainly not admissible to "overlook" these pathologies. A subsequent sequence (ideally axial T1-weighted) through the neck, thorax, abdomen, and pelvis can be additionally supplemented to avoid having to call back the volunteers for a second exam in this not inconsiderable percentage of cases. Nowadays this sequence should be three dimensional, on the one hand for reasons of good image quality with an adequate signal-to-noise ratio while still maintaining a small slice thickness, and on the other hand for the option of multiplanar image reconstruction. For similar reasons, the entire examination should be followed by a T1 sequence of the head, which should be performed as a contrast-enhanced sequence following the preceding administration of contrast agent to detect less common, but relevant, cerebral tumors more reliably.

What these incidental results ultimately means to the volunteer, whether the discovery of some benign or malignant disease positively influences his life and well-being in the long term, is still unclear. The answer to this question is particularly complicated by the diversity of diseases that can be diagnosed in MRI and the nontrivial combination of effects on the volunteer.

12.5   Decision-making strategies

Screening with MRI is really very much in its infancy. Studies have to clarify some questions before partial or whole-body screening should be actively recommended.

12.5.1   Diagnostic accuracy and predictive value

The diagnostic accuracy of whole-body MR strategies is largely known from individual clinical examinations, and, insofar as the same protocols are used, these are theoretically transferable to whole-body screening examinations, as long as no compromises in the image quality and number of sequences are made.

Positive and negative predictive values are crucial parameters for the quality and "meaningfulness" of a screening test; these are strongly dependent on the collectives studied and cannot simply be extrapolated from previous clinical studies of discrete diseases. From the clinical perspective, we consider the outcome of symptomatic persons with known diseases; from the screening perspective, we mainly consider healthy, non-symptomatic persons. Ideally we would have knowledge of the positive and negative predictive values for all individual detectable diseases. As long as these are not accurately known, screening should primarily be performed for diseases that appear suitable for this purpose on the basis of previous experience.

12.5.2   Unresolved questions

We have to admit that we have hardly any concrete knowledge on the cost-benefit ratio of such examinations, especially when it comes to non-focused whole-body MRI examinations, which underlines the necessity of prospective large-scale studies. These should be conducted under controlled conditions and should include both defined patient and volunteer selection as well as long-term documentation of the benefit for the studied group, which ultimately has to be weighed against the cost for the individual and the general public.

The low number of relevant results in a "normal collective" as in [86] at least leads to the speculation that the total cost-benefit effect of such complex techniques as a 60-minute MR whole-body examination would not be economically justifiable overall. In the future it is above all a matter of conducting preselection to raise the prevalence and thereby the cost-effectiveness of a whole-body MRI. A very promising group for whole-body atherosclerosis screening is formed for example by CHD patients, who in up to 50% of cases show renal artery stenoses or carotid stenoses. The individual has a different perspective, as shown by the growing number of self-referrers, and not only if the early detection of – uncommon – relevant diseases leads to a prolongation of life or simply to an enhancement in quality of life. For the individual, even a negative result can represent a major positive value, which is hard to measure in monetary terms.

Other important factors still to be clarified before MRI is offered as a screening technique pertain to the availability of suitable systems; the costs for any supplementary and invasive investigations; the morbidity and mortality rates in case of false-negative results, but positive results as well; the psychological implications both of negative and of positive results; the subsequent support for the patient by the relevant specialists; and many more besides. And before the health insurance companies even consider accepting the costs, the cost-benefit effect also has to be clarified. An important measure for the benefit of medical measures in general, which should also be applied here, is the term "QUALY" (quality-adjusted life years), whose determination depends on repeated extensive surveys on physical and psychological health and well-being.

12.5.3   Volunteer support and information

Because the implications of such whole-body screening examinations, which have only recently been available, are not yet known, the requestors, whether they are referring physicians or self-referrers, should be informed in particular detail of all possible advantages and disadvantages. Here it is above all important that the radiologist explains the limitations of the technique in order that the volunteer is not convinced that they are "completely" healthy in the case of a negative result. MRI simply allows the diagnosis of diseases ultimately accompanied by morphological changes. The conclusiveness of vascular changes must also be discussed: In the case of non-significant stenoses, the luminography of the carotid alone does not permit the conclusion that there is no risk of stroke, because the condition of the vessel walls, which are not studied in most screening protocols, plays a particularly important role; it must also be mentioned that the heart examination still usually shows a low sensitivity for the detection of CHD, especially in its early stages.

The limitations of many whole-body examinations often include the inability to assess entire organs, such as the breast, prostate, or the small intestine for instance. The radiologist must fulfill his/her role as a physician with his/her knowledge extending beyond radiology, understand the expectations of the patients with regard to the planned screening test, and inform the volunteer of alternative diagnostic tests as applicable (diabetes mellitus, for example, is still diagnosed today with a simple glucose tolerance test).

The long-term effects of secondary results on the quality of life of the volunteers have been investigated to an even lesser degree; the simple extrapolation of clinical study results to healthy volunteers is not possible.

12.6   MR screening in the future

12.6.1   System developments

The system manufacturers have recognized contemporary demands and have reacted with system developments that not only accelerate data acquisition and computation (the current buzzword is "parallel imaging" even for whole-body imaging [88, 89] (also see Chap. 1), but also include table movement and the effective use of dedicated coils. These developments have led to an entirely new way of thinking about and using MRI systems. The possibilities offered by whole-body examinations, whether for detection of tumors and metastases or of vascular changes, have already led to a diagnostic paradigm shift, at least in the larger radiological centers. On the one hand, tertiary "screening" can be performed in a single MRI examination depending on the tumor type (see Chap. 6, 7, and 8); on the other, the readiness to participate in such extensive secondary prevention screening measures has increased markedly, even though the costs are initially borne personally. Continued rapid development, especially in the field of radio frequency technology and pulse sequence design, is set to further simplify MRI screening and make it less expensive at the same time. For these reasons, MRI screening examinations will increasingly be the focus of scientific and commercial interest.

12.6.2   New indications

One of the greatest challenges is without doubt the reliable and accurate imaging of the coronary arteries. This addition would incorporate a measure of the most important cause of death in a comprehensive assessment. In the field of malignant diseases, the ability to assess the lung parenchyma must in particular be improved.

MRI as a screening technique for the diagnosis of colonic lesions, especially of the precursors and entities concurrent with a colon carcinoma, appears to already offer sufficient diagnostic reliability.

12.6.3   Paradigm shift in secondary prevention?

Before MR screening can be offered on a large scale, prospective studies ultimately have to clarify the relationship between the benefit for the examinee and the costs they and the general population incur. But even before the relevant results are available, it would appear probable that MRI will play a crucial role in the increasingly prominent field of secondary prevention. This is due to the fact that the majority of relevant diseases, such as malignant tumors and vascular diseases, can be detected at a very early stage with MRI. At the same time, we are sure to see a shift in diagnostic measures from clinical departments towards radiology (established examples include whole-body angiography for planning the therapy of patients with arterial pathologies, as well as the diagnosis of colonic pathologies). As is already recognizable today, individuals will increasingly present themselves of their own initiative to radiology to obtain a check up. In this situation, the radiologist often adopts the role of a navigator, who, like the patient's primary care physician, has to advise on further diagnostic and therapeutic measures in case of a positive result. Whole-body MRI screening is certain to bestow an increasing number of examinations on radiology in the future, but also to impose new responsibilities upon the radiologist.

Bibliography

1. Lerman C, Trock Brimer BK, Boyce A, Jepson C, Engstrom PF. Psychological and behavioral implications of abnormal mammograms. Ann Int Med 1991; 114: 657–61.

2. Cordes L, Heine F, Krickau G. Results of mass radiography for tuberculosis in older school children. Offentl Gesundheitswes 1972; 34: 173–9.

3. Olivotto IA, Kan L, d'Yachkova Y, et al. Ten years of breast screening in the Screening Mammography Program of British Columbia, 1988–1997. J Med Screen 2000; 7(3): 152–9.

4. Nystrom L, Andersson I, Bjurstam N, Frisell J, Nordenskjold B, Rutqvist LE. Long-term effects of mammography screening: updated overview of the Swedish andomized trials. Lancet 2002; 359(9310): 909–19.

5. Gotzsche PC, Olsen O. Is screening for breast cancer with mammography justifiable? Lancet 2000; 355(9198): 129–34.

6. Kopp AF, Schroeder S, Baumbach A, Kuettner A, Georg C, Ohnesorge B, Heuschmid M, Kuzo R, Claussen CD. Non-invasive haracterization of coronary lesion morphology and composition by multislice CT: first results in comparison with intracoronary ultrasound. Eur Radiol 2001; 11(9): 1607–11.

7. Henschke CI, McCauley DI, Yankelevitz DF, et al. Early Lung Cancer Action Project: overall design and findings from baseline screening. Lancet 1999; 354: 99–105.

8. Diederich S, Wormanns D, Semik M, et al. Screening for early lung cancer with low-dose spiral CT: prevalence in 817 asymptomatic smokers. Radiology 2002; 222: 773–8.

9. Johnson CD, Dachman AH. CT colonography: the next colon screening examination? Radiology 2000; 216(2): 331–41.

10. Elsberry RB. The invasion of the body scanner. Decisions in imaging economics. February 2002. Available at: http://www.imagingeconomics.com/library/200202-03.asp. Zugänglich im Mai 2005.

11. United States Center for Food and Drug Administration. Whole body scanning: using computed tomography (CT). Center for Devices and Radiological Health. April 17, 2002. http://www.fda.gov/cdrh/ct/. Zugänglich im Mai 2005.

12. Reducing Radiation Risk from Computed Tomography for Pediatric and Small Adult Patients. In: Safety Alerts, Public Health Advisories and Notices from CDRH. FDA Notice 11/2/2001.

13. Kalish GM, Bhargavan M, Sunshine JH, Forman HP. Self-referred whole-body imaging: where are we now? Radiology 2004; 233(2): 353–8.

14. Stellungnahme des Bundesministeriums für Umwelt, Naturschutz und Reaktorsicherheit (BMU) (2002). www.kvbb.de/jsp/epctrl.jsp. Zugänglich Mai 2005.

15. Bekanntmachung der Kassenärztlichen Bundesvereinigung (2004). Beschluss einer Änderung der Richtlinien des Bundesausschusses der Ärzte und Krankenkassen über die Früherkennung von Krebserkrankungen („Krebsfrüherkennungs-Richtlinien") in der Fassung vom 26. April 1976 vom 15.12.2003. Dtsch Ärztebl 6: 289.

16. Frisell J, Lidbrink E, Hellstrom L, Rutqvist LE. Follow-up after 11 years: update of mortality results in the Stockholm mammographic screening trial. Breast Cancer Res Treat 1997; 45: 263–270.

17. European Reference Organisation for Quality Assured Breast Screening and Diagnostic Service (EUREF). European Guidelines for Qualitiy Assurance in Mammography Screening. Third edition, European Communities, January 2001.

18. Perry N, Broeders M, de Wolf C, Törnberg S (eds). European guidelines for quality assurance in mammography screening. 3rd edn. European Communities, Luxemburg, 2001.

19. BMU-Hintergrundpapier Stand: 28. Januar 2004. http://www.bmu.de/files/pdfs/allgemein/application/pdf/ammography_screenings.pdf. Zugänglich Mai 2005.

20. Budinger TF. MR safety: past, present, and future from a historical perspective. Magn Reson Imaging Clin N Am. 1998; 6(4): 701–14.

21. Prince MR, Arnoldus C, Frisoli JK. Nephrotoxicity of high-dose gadolinium compared with iodinated contrast. J Magn Reson Imaging 1996; 6162–66.

22. Shellock FG, Kanal E. Safety of magnetic resonance imaging contrast agents. J Magn Reson Imaging 1999; 10: 477–84.

23. Tombach B, Bremer C, Reimer P, et al. Renal tolerance of a neutral gadolinium chelate (gadobutrol) in patients with chronic renal failure: results of a randomized study. Radiology 2001; 218: 651–7.

24. Li F, Sone S, Maruyama Y, et al. Correlation between high-resolution computed tomographic, magnetic resonance and pathological findings in cases with non-cancerous but suspicious lung nodules. Eur Radiol 2000; 10(11): 1782–91.

25. Chung MH, Lee HG, Kwon SS, Park SH. MR imaging of solitary pulmonary lesions: emphasis on tuberculomas and comparison with tumors. J Magn Reson Imaging 2000; 11(6): 629–37.

26. Engelbrecht MR, Huisman HJ, Laheij RJ, et al. Discrimination of prostate cancer from normal peripheral zone and central gland tissue by using dynamic contrast-enhanced MR imaging. Radiology 2003; 229(1): 248–54.

27. Cornud F, Flam T, Chauveinc L, et al. Extraprostatic spread of clinically localized prostate cancer: factors predictive of pT3 tumor and of positive endorectal MR imaging examination results. Radiology 2002; 224: 203–10.

28. Crowe JP, Gordon NH, Shenk RR, Zollinger RM, Brumberg DJ, Shuck JM. Primary tumor size: relevance to breast cancer survival. Arch Surg 1992; 127: 910–5.

29. Kawashima H, Matsui O, Suzuki M, et al. Breast cancer in dense breast: detection with contrast-enhanced dynamic MR imaging. J Magn Reson Imaging 2000; 11: 233–43.

30. Kuhl CK, Schmutzler RK, Leutner CC, et al. Breast MR imaging screening in 192 women proved or suspected to be carriers of a breast cancer susceptibility gene: preliminary results. Radiology 2000; 215: 267–79.

31. Weinreb JC, Newstead G. MR imaging of the breast. Radiology 1995;196: 593–610.

32. Neuhaus H. Screening for colorectal cancer in Germany: guidelines and reality. Endoscopy 1999; 31(6): 468–70.

33. O'Brien MJ, Winawer SJ, Zauber AG, et al. The National Polyp Study. Patient and polyp characteristics associated with high-grade dysplasia in colorectal adenomas. Gastroenterology 1990; 98: 371–9.

34. Liebermann DA, Smith FW. Screening for colon malignancy with colonoscopy. Am J Gastroenterol 1991; 86: 946–51.

35. Landis SH, Murray T, Bodden S , Wingo PA. Cancer statistics 1998. CA Cancer J Clin 1998; 48: 6–29.

36. Luboldt W, Bauerfeind P, Steiner P, Fried M, Krestin GP, Debatin J. Preliminary assessment of three-dimensional magnetic resonance imaging for various colonic disorder. Lancet 1997; 349: 1288–91.

37. Fenlon HM, Nunes DP, Schroy PC, et al. A comparison of virtual and conventional colonoscopy for the detection of colorectal polyps. N Engl J Med 1999; 341: 1496–503.

38. Pappalardo G, Polettini E, Frattaroli FM, et al. Magnetic resonance colonography versus conventional colonoscopy for the detection of colonic endoluminal lesions. Gastroenterology 2000; 119: 300–4.

39. Saar B, Heverhagen JT, Obst T, et al. Magnetic resonance colonography and virtual magnetic resonance colonoscopy with the 1.0-T system: a feasibility study. Invest Radiol 2000; 35: 521–6.

40. Villavicencio RT, Rex DX. Colonic adenomas: prevalence and incidence rates, growth rates, and miss rates at colonoscopy. Semin Gastrointest Dis 2000; 11: 185–93.

41. Lauenstein TC, Debatin JF. Magnetic resonance colonography for colorectal cancer screening. Semin Ultrasound CT MR 2001; 22: 443–53.

42. Lauenstein TC, Goehde SC, Ruehm SG, Holtmann G, Debatin JF. MR colonography with barium-based fecal tagging: initial clinical experience. Radiology 2002; 223: 248–54.

43. Smith PA, Fishman EK. Clinical integration of three-dimensional helical CT angiography into academic radiology: results of a focused survey. AJR Am J Roentgenol 1999; 173(2): 445–7.

44. Nederkoorn PJ, Mali WP, Eikelboom BC, et al. Preoperative diagnosis of carotid artery stenosis: accuracy of noninvasive testing. Stroke 2002; 33(8): 2003–8.

45. Korst MB, Joosten FB, Postma CT, Jager GJ, Krabbe JK, Barentsz JO. Accuracy of normal-dose contrast-enhanced MR angiography in assessing renal artery stenosis and accessory renal arteries. AJR Am J Roentgenol 2000; 174(3): 629–34.

46. Hany TF, Debatin JF, Leung DA, Pfammatter T. Evaluation of the aortoiliac and renal arteries: comparison of breath-hold, contrast-enhanced, three-dimensional MR angiography with conventional catheter angiography. Radiology 1997; 204(2): 357–62.

47. Meaney JF, Ridgway JP, Chakraverty S, et al. Stepping-table gadolinium-enhanced digital subtraction MR angiography of the aorta and lower extremity arteries: preliminary experience. Radiology 1999; 211: 59–67.

48. Ho KY, Leiner T, de Haan MW, et al. Peripheral vascular tree stenoses: evaluation with moving-bed infusion-tracking MR angiography. Radiology 1998; 206: 683–92.

49. Ruehm SG, Hany TF, Pfammatter T, et al. Pelvic and lower extremity arterial imaging: diagnostic performance of three-dimensional contrast-enhanced MR angiography. Am J Roentgenol 2000; 174: 1127–35.

50. Goyen M, Quick HH, Debatin JF, et al. Whole body 3D MR angiography using a rolling table platform: initial clinical experience. Radiology 2002; 224: 270–7.

51. Fenchel M, Requardt M, Tomaschko K, et al. Whole-body MR angiography using a novel 32-receiving-channel MR system with surface coil technology: first clinical experience. J Magn Reson Imaging. 2005; 21(5): 596–603.

52. Anderson KM, Wilson PWF, Odell PM, Kannel WB. An updated coronary risk profile: a statement for health professionals. Circulation 1991; 83: 356–62.

53. Barkhausen J, Ruehm SG, Goyen M, Buck T, Laub G, Debatin JF. MR evaluation of ventricular function: true fast imaging with steady-state precession versus fast low-angle shot cine MR imaging: feasibility study. Radiology 2001; 219: 264–9.

54. Van der Geest RJ, Reiber JHC. Quantification in cardiac MRI. JMRI 1999; 10: 602–8.

55. Friedrich MG, Schulz-Menger J, Poetsch T, Pilz B, Uhlich F, Dietz R. Quantification of valvular aortic stenosis by magnetic resonance imaging. Am Heart J 2002; 144: 329–34.

56. Canet EP, Janier MF, Revel D. Magnetic resonance perfusion imaging in ischemic heart disease. J Magn Reson Imaging 1999; 10: 423–33.

57. Wilke NM, Jerosch-Herold M, Zenovich A, et al. Magnetic resonance first-pass myocardial perfusion imaging: clinical validation and future applications. J Magn Reson Imaging 1999; 10: 676–85.

58. Pereira RS, Wisenberg G, Prato FS, Yvorchuk K. Clinical assessment of myocardial viability using MRI during a constant infusion of Gd-DTPA. MAGMA 2000; 11(3): 104–13.

59. Hunold P, Brandt-Mainz K, Freudenberg L, et al. Evaluation of myocardial viability with contrast-enhanced magnetic resonance imaging – comparison of the late enhancement technique with positron emission tomography. Rofo Fortschr Geb Rontgenstr Neuen Bildgeb Verfahr 2002; 174(7): 867–73.

60. Giang TH, Nanz D, Coulden R, et al. Detection of coronary artery disease by magnetic resonance myocardial perfusion imaging with various contrast agent doses: first European multi-center experience. Eur Heart J 2004; 25(18): 1657–65.

61. Hirai T, Korogi Y, Ono K, Nagano M, Maruoka K, Uemura S, Takahashi M. Prospective evaluation of suspected stenoocclusive disease of the intracranial artery: combined MR angiography and CT angiography compared with digital subtraction angiography. AJNR Am J Neuroradiol 2002; 23: 93–101.

62. Herskovits EH, Itoh R, Melhem ER. Accuracy for detection of simulated lesions: comparison of fluid-attenuated inversion-recovery, proton density-weighted, and T2-weighted synthetic brain MR imaging. AJR Am J Roentgenol 2001; 176: 1313–8.

63. Kim DE, Bae HJ, Lee SH, Kim H, Yoon BW, Roh JK. Gradient echo magnetic resonance imaging in the prediction of hemorrhagic vs ischemic stroke: a need for the consideration of the extent of leukoariosis. Arch Neurol 2002; 59: 425–9.

64. Blake LM, Scheinman MM, Higgins CB. MR features of arrhythmogenic right ventricular dysplasia. AJR Am J Roentgenol 1994; 162: 809–12.

65. Vignaux O, Lazarus A, Varin J, et al. Right ventricular MR abnormalities in myotonic dystrophy and relationship with intracardiac electrophysiologic test findings: initial results. Radiology 2002; 224: 231–5.

66. Ruehm SG, Wiesner W, Debatin JF. Pelvic and lower extremity veins: contrast-enhanced three-dimensional MR venography with a dedicated vascular coil-initial experience. Radiology 2000; 215(2): 421–7.

67. Wilhelm Poll L, Wittsack HJ, Koch JA, et al. A rapid and reliable semiautomated method for measurement of total abdominal fat volumes using magnetic resonance imaging. Magn Reson Imaging 2003; 21(6): 631–6.

68. Shen W, Punyanitya M, Wang Z, et al. Total body skeletal muscle and adipose tissue volumes: estimation from a single abdominal cross-sectional image. J Appl Physiol. 2004; 97: 2333–8.

69. Abe T, Kojima K, Kearns CF, Yohena H, Fukuda J. Whole body muscle hypertrophy from resistance training: distribution and total mass. Br Sports Med 2003; 37: 543–5.

70. Liu KH, Chan YL, Chan WB, Kong WL, Kong MO, Chan JC. Sonographic measurement of mesenteric fat thickness is a good correlate with cardiovascular risk factors: comparison with subcutaneous and preperitoneal fat thickness, magnetic resonance imaging and anthropometric indexes. Int J Obes Relat Metab Disord 2003; 27(10): 1267–73.

71. Ryan M, Twair A, Nelson E, Brennan D, Eustace S. Whole body magnetic resonance imaging in the diagnosis of Parsonage Turner syndrome. Acta Radiol 2004; 45(5): 534–9.

72. Lenk S, Fischer S, Kotter I, Claussen CD, Schlemmer HP. [Possibilities of whole-body MRI for investigating musculoskeletal diseases]. Radiologe 2004; 44(9): 844–53.

73. Pichiecchio A, Uggetti C, Egitto MG, et al. Quantitative MR evaluation of body composition in patients with Duchenne muscular dystrophy. Eur Radiol 2002; 12(11): 2704–9.

74. Wedegartner U, Tchirikov M, Koch M, et al. Functional magnetic resonance imaging (fMRI) for fetal oxygenation during maternal hypoxia: initial results. Rofo Fortschr Geb Rontgenstr Neuen Bildgeb Verfahr 2002; 174: 700–3.

75. Levine D, Zuo C, Faro CB, Chen Q. Potential heating effect in the gravid uterus during MR HASTE imaging. J Magn Reson Imaging 2001; 13(6): 856–61.

76. Narra VR, Howell RW, Goddu SM, Rao DV. Effects of a 1.5-Tesla static magnetic field on spermatogenesis and embryogenesis in mice. Invest Radiol. 1996; 31(9): 586–90.

77. Rofsky NM, Pizzarello DJ, Weinreb JC, Ambrosino MM, Rosenberg C. Effect on fetal mouse development of exposure to MR imaging and gadopentetate dimeglumine. J Magn Reson Imaging 1994; 4(6): 805–7.

78. Chew S, Ahmadi A, Goh PS, Foong LC. The effects of 1.5T magnetic resonance imaging on early murine in-vitro embryo development. J Magn Reson Imaging 2001; 13(3): 417–20.

79. Klop RB, Eikelboom BC, Taks AC, et al. Screening of the internal carotid arteries in patients with peripheral vascular disease by colour-flow duplex scanning. Eur J Vasc Surg 1991; 5: 41–5.

80. Alexandrova NA, Gibson WC, Norris JW, Maggisano R: Carotid artery stenosis in peripheral vascular disease. J Vasc Surg 1996; 23: 645–9.

81. McDaniel MD, Cronenwett JL. Basic data related to the natural history of intermittent claudication. Ann Vasc Surg 1989; 3: 273–7.

82. Lundblad D, Eliasson M. Silent myocardial infarction in women with impaired glucose tolerance: The Northern Sweden MONICA study. Cardiovasc Diabetol 2003; 2(1): 9.

83. Gohde SC, Goyen M, Forsting M, Debatin JF. Prevention without radiation – a strategy for comprehensive early detection using magnetic resonance imaging. Radiologe 2002; 42(8): 622–9.

84. Vogt FM, Herborn CU, Hunold P, Lauenstein TC, Schroder T, Debatin JF, Barkhausen J. HASTE MRI versus chest radiography in the detection of pulmonary nodules: comparison with MDCT. AJR Am J Roentgenol 2004; 183(1): 71–8.

85. Ajaj W, Pelster G, Treichel U, Vogt FM, Debatin JF, Ruehm SG, Lauenstein TC. Dark lumen magnetic resonance colonography: comparison with conventional colonoscopy for the detection of colorectal pathology. Gut 2003; 52(12): 1738–43.

86. Goehde SC, Hunold P, Vogt FM, et al. Full-body cardiovascular and tumor MRI for early detection of disease: feasibility and initial experience in 298 subjects. AJR Am J Roentgenol. 2005; 184(2): 598–611.

87. Hawighorst H, Schoenberg SO, Knopp MV, Essig M, Miltner P, van Kaick G. Hepatic lesions: morphologic and functional characterization with multiphase breath-hold 3D gadolinium-enhanced MR angiography – initial results. Radiology 1999; 210: 89–96.

88. Kramer H, Schoenberg SO, Nikolaou K. [Cardiovascular whole body MRI with parallel imaging]. Radiologe 2004; 44(9): 835–43.

89. Quick HH, Vogt FM, Maderwald S, Herborn CU, Bosk S, Gohde S, Debatin JF, Ladd ME. High spatial resolution whole-body MR angiography featuring parallel imaging: initial experience. Rofo 2004; 176(2): 163–9.

13 Virtual autopsy in forensic science using MRI – initial experiences

Michael Thali

Since the discovery of X-rays by Wilhelm C. Röntgen in 1895, they have found use in many radioscopic technology applications. At that time, not even a year passed before postmortem examinations on mummies and the deceased had been performed [1]. Today, photographs of the first postmortem X-ray recordings from 1898 can be marveled at in radiological museums in the USA [1]. Ultrasound technology, which was introduced a few decades later, has also been used for postmortem examinations [2]. And in the 1970s, computed tomography (CT) arrived for postmortem examinations. Pioneer work was carried out by Bratzke et al. in 1982, which indicated that the postmortem CT could possibly play a role regarding the ban on autopsy [3]. The idea of postmortem examinations of gunshot injuries using CT was first proposed by Clasen and Torack in 1982 [4]. From 1983 onwards, Schumacher et al. published their work on the subject of "computed tomographic examinations of wound ballistics of cranial gunshot injuries" in which intravital CT gunshot injury examination results were compared with neuropathological sections [5, 6]. They arrived at the conclusion that imaging methods such as CT are a valuable addition to neuropathological examinations in forensic investigations and could even be effectively used prior to general neuropathological processing of the prepared brain. Their work also showed that CT technology, which had just been introduced at the time, could differentiate between entry and exit wounds, as well as allow the course of the shot channel to be depicted. After spiral tomography was introduced in 1989 by Willi Kalender from Erlangen and Peter Vock from Berne on the occasion of the RSNA Conference in Chicago, three dimensional imaging of the body was successful for the first time [7]. This surmounted the limitations of 2D images with three-dimensional body geometry, and the era of 3D visualization had also begun for forensic science.

As CT is the slice imaging technique of choice for bony structures and pathological gas accumulations, yet shows significant weaknesses in soft tissue structures, magnetic resonance imaging (MRI) is gaining in importance, also in postmortem applications [8–18]. MRI can plug precisely the gaps that CT has hitherto left open.

Its utilization in the field of forensic medicine began with a case published by Amberg in 1989 regarding the identification of a deceased person performed by magnetic resonance imaging [19]. Thereafter, MRI was mainly used for postmortem examinations of fetuses and infants. The first comparative study was conducted in 1990 by Ross et al., in which the examination results of six cases were compared between postmortem MRI and autopsy [20]. Numerous postmortem MR studies on fetuses followed [21–23]. Only towards the end of the 1990s were isolated research groups successful in overcoming the organizational and logistical hurdles for postmortem imaging of human corpses with MRI, as until this time it was only possible to scan using systems in the clinic outside of the patient care schedule [10–13, 16].

During this period, the Institute of Forensic Medicine at the University of Berne, Switzerland, under the leadership of Prof. Dr. med. Richard Dirnhofer, shifted its research focus towards the field of forensic imaging. The institute had been involved for many years with 3-dimensional surface documentation [24–29]. Modern tomographic imaging techniques were designed to facilitate non-invasive imaging beneath the surface of the body, and thus the methods of 3D body surface documentation were supplemented with radiological imaging by means of CT and MRI. The aim was to produce a fused data set from surface documentation and volume scanning of the human corpse, which could be used to carry out at any time a virtual autopsy to clarify questions arising in the sense of a "forensically visible human". The research project implemented in Berne was initially termed "Scalpel-free Autopsy" or "Digital Autopsy", but was then renamed to the now trademarked "VIRTOPSY", indicating image-guided minimal-invasive autopsy.

The pseudonym VIRTOPSY is composed of the two words "virtual" and "autopsy" [16]:
• "virtual" originates from Latin and stands for virtuous and
• "autopsy" means "to see with one's own eyes".

The Institute for Forensic Medicine at the University of Berne, in collaboration with the Diagnostic Institute for Radiology and Neuroradiology at the University Hospital of Berne, decided to systematically evaluate the new tomographic techniques of CT and MRI for the forensic sciences and to adapt them for postmortem use.

The challenge of the radiological part of the VIRTOPSY project is to develop through suitable cases an image-guided, minimally-invasive autopsy to supplement the classical autopsy technique, so that opening up the corpse in forensic science can be partially or in some cases completely avoided [16, 30–33]. The autopsies takes place virtually on the radiological tomographic data set; the objective results can be documented two or three dimensionally independent of the examiner and further analyzed in this form and vividly demonstrated to the courts using 2D or 3D reconstructions.

Over the years, the previous VIRTOPSY technologies (3D surface scanning, postmortem CT and MRI) were supplemented with microradiological examinations (micro CT and micro MR) as well as magnetic resonance spectroscopy [34, 35]. In 2004, the methods were also supplemented with postmortem image-guided biopsy to obtain fluids for chemical-toxicological analyses, as well as for microscopic examinations. The first postmortem minimally-invasive angiographies were also performed [36]. In this way, an autopsy case can be assessed from its macroscopic (including angiological), histological, and toxicological aspects.

Part of the VIRTOPSY project is intended to evaluate whether the points of relevance for the forensic medicine expert report, such as cause of death or atrium mortis, as well as the pathomorphological results in the soft tissue, bone, and organ structures, can be assessed and documented using imaging.

The Institute for Forensic Medicine of the University has investigated 120 postmortem cases so far using whole-body CT and whole-body MRI. The radiological examination was accompanied with a classical postmortem autopsy in each case. This allows the accurately detailed correlation of radiological data with those from the autopsy and thus comparative post-processing of the forensic results as are presented by the Armed Forces Institute of Pathology (AFIP) in the field of clinical pathology.

The MRI examinations have taken place with a 1.5 Tesla MRI system up till now. All regions of the body were examined in each case. The complete examination of a complex traffic accident, for example, entails an examination time of 2–3 h.

With regard to cause of death, MRI examinations are particularly well suited for detecting brain trauma and brain damage (Figs. 13.1, 13.2, 13.10). In some cases it can provide supplementary information to the autopsy if intracranial hemorrhaging drains away during the autopsy and is then difficult to assess in its localization and extent.

Edematous findings can also be significantly better delineated in the MRI than macroscopically during the autopsy of the organ (Fig. 13.10). The cerebral structures of brain regions subject to severe decomposition are also shown in the MRI and can still be intracranially assessed, which, during the autopsy, can only be identified as brain tissue debris and cannot be macroscopically diagnosed.

The use of MRI in the cardiovascular system is of importance. Although coronary calcification can only be assessed with difficulty in the CT in regard to its contribution as a cause of death, MRI provides the possibility of also diagnosing myocardial changes.

It was possible to identify cardiac infarctions comparable with autopsy, as long as they had been survived for at least a few hours (Fig. 13.7). The subsequent infarct healing stages are clearly conspicuous in the postmortem cardiac MRI on account of their vital reactions. The collagen infarct scars, as ultimate residues of myocardial ischemias, are clearly apparent in the postmortem MRI. Coronary constrictions and closures can be diagnosed with contrast agent CT and related to myocardial changes to complete cardiac diagnostics [36].

In the lung examination, inner livor mortis in the posterior regions, which can be misinterpreted as pneumonias by radiologists not familiar with postmortem imaging, are particularly conspicuous. A pneumothorax is also clearly identifiable in postmortem imaging; however, although post-traumatic lung contusions and blood aspiration lesions may indeed be diagnosed, they are difficult to distinguish from one another in the individual case [16].

Ideally, the visualization and diagnosis of traumatic results in the skeletal system in CT can be supplemented with MRI to present the corresponding soft tissue injuries in the fatty tissue and in the muscular system, which is of crucial importance in reconstructive inves-

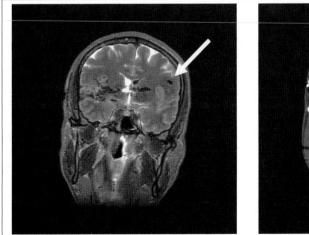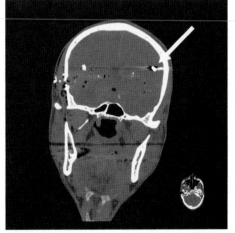

Figure 13.1 Suicidal shot to the head. Shot channel in MRI (coronal T2, left) and in the corresponding orientation in CT (right): subcutaneous hemorrhaging right temporal (hyperdense); hypointense and hypodense gas and hyperdense hemorrhaging in the shot channel; projectile fragment frontal left (arrow) with signal loss in MRI and streaking artifacts in CT.

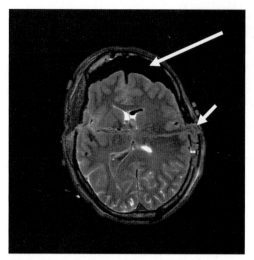

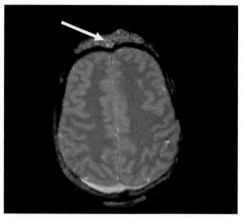

Figure 13.3 Burned corpse with serious charring. Fire hematoma (arrow): brain axial, GRASS sequence (T2-weighting), frontal epidural, crescent-shaped, inhomogeneous hyperintense volume displacement between tabula interna of the calvaria and dura mater, typical for a fire hematoma. Subdural semi-circular gas accumulation caused by heat-related intracranial vapor pressure (black in the image), occipital fluid level.

Figure 13.2 Suicidal shot through the head. Shot channel in the MRI: temporo-frontal course of the shot channel with the escape of brain tissue left temporal (short arrow), crescent-shaped frontal pneumocephalus (longer arrow).

tigations in forensic medicine [17]. The method of choice is MRI, not least due to its significantly higher soft tissue contrast, although larger lesions are also detectable in CT examinations [37]. Whereas the diagnosis of brain damage presents no major problems, the examination of traumatic lesions is difficult, above all in the liver, if death occurred suddenly and only small pathological blood accumulations or none at all could form in the region of the lesion.

Heart wall injuries, whether traumatic or post-infarct, are far easier to ascertain, alone by the subsequent pericardial tamponade. The most important forensic vital reactions, such as air or gas embolisms, can be diagnosed without difficulties. Additional important vital indications, such as fat embolisms, i.e. an influx of minute fat particles from contusions of fatty tissue regions or bone fractures into the lung, cannot as yet be clearly depicted radiologically.

Tomographic imaging is ideal for visualization and subsequent forensic reconstruction of injury results, especially with the improved comprehensibility for the medical laymen of the criminal justice system and law enforcement. The improved comprehensibility of medical results for those without medical training naturally leads to closer and more effective collaboration. The 3D presentations from CT were the first to leave a decisive impression on the investigating authorities.

During the VIRTOPSY project, several cases of strangulation were investigated by comparing postmortem images and autopsies. These results are now being used in the examination of victims who have survived suffocation or strangulation to assess the level of violence applied against the neck [38]. Until now, only the anamnesis and the externally visible cutaneous injuries could be drawn upon, as invasive diagnostics without a medical

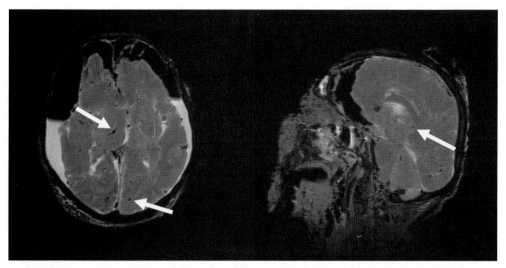

Figure 13.4 Decayed corpse after 13 months in water. Advanced decay of the brain tissue: T2 axial (left) and sagittal (right) deformed and compressed brain with isolated intracerebral gas bubbles (arrow), as well as crescent-shaped subdural accumulations of gas under the calvaria, hyperintense subdural fluid accumulations, and relatively well preserved intracerebral structures.

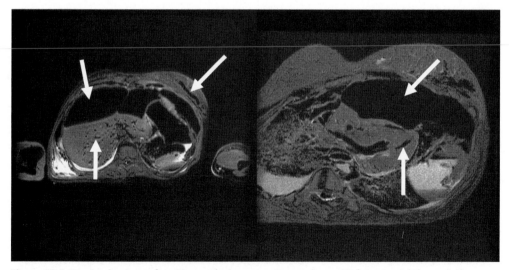

Figure 13.5 Decayed corpse after 13 months in water. Organ decay: T2 fat sat axial through the upper abdomen (left) and thorax (right) with accumulations of putrefaction gas (arrows): intraperitoneal, intrahepatic, subcutaneous, intramyocardial, intrathoracic. Accumulations of putrefaction fluid: intrathoracic as pleural effusion.

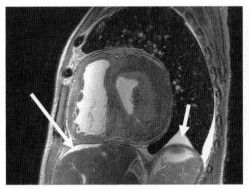

Figure 13.6 Natural death due to cardiac insufficiency.

Cor bovinum: short axis slice through right and left heart chambers, extreme biventricular eccentric hypertrophied heart.

Pleural effusion dorsal (short arrow) and some ascites over the liver (long arrow) as signal-intense fluid accumulations.

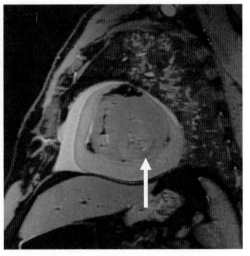

Figure 13.7 Natural death due to cardiac infarction.

Cardiac infarct rear wall (arrow): short axis slice, STIR sequence, hypointense crescent-shaped infarct region with minimal hyperintense edematous margin. Subsequent pericardial tamponade with partially coagulated and partly fluid hyperintense blood.

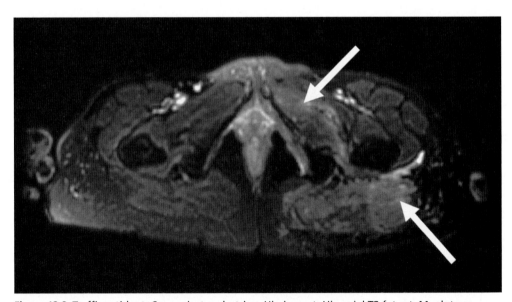

Figure 13.8 Traffic accident: Car against pedestrian. Hip impact: Hip axial T2 fat sat. M. gluteus maximus and M. adductor magnus left diffuse hyperintense and swollen, consistent with an edema (arrow). Additional minimal edematous dorsal swelling of subcutaneous fat tissue of M. gluteus maximus left.

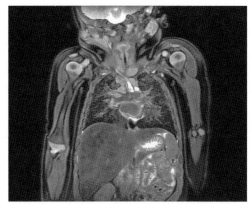

Figure 13.9 SIDS (sudden infant death syndrome). Coronal, T2 fat sat of normal neck, thorax, and abdomen: section includes trachea, pulmonary vessels, left atrium, lungs, liver, spleen, and stomach.

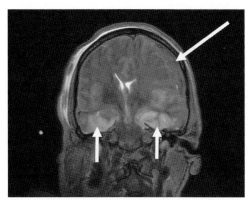

Figure 13.10 Fall on the head. Coronal slice orientation, T2: subgaleal hyperintensity right (coup) with subsequent subdural hemorrhage (longer arrow) left (contre coup). Basal brain infarcts temporal bilateral (short arrow) with increased intracranial pressure.

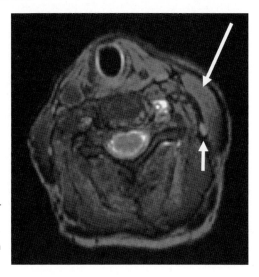

Figure 13.11 Death by strangulation. Axial slice orientation, T2: The left M. sternocleidomastoideus (longer arrow) is significantly more signal-intense than contralaterally, and swollen, signal-intense lymph nodes are conspicuous ipsilaterally in the internal structures (short arrow).

indication for the assessment of the case are not permitted. Through the use of MRI in clinical forensic medicine, results ascertained by autopsy of deeper structures in the neck can be used for the forensic assessment of living victims.

The VIRTOPSY project is conducted under the leadership of the Institute for Forensic Medicine in close cooperation with the general and neuroradiological departments of the University Hospital in Berne, as well as the Department for Magnetic Resonance Spectroscopy and Methodology. Further collaborations exist between national and international partners (www.virtopsy.com). Several examples from the forensic case collection have been selected (c.f. figures), which represent rather unusual entities for the clinical radiologist.

- Hip impact
- Fire hematoma
- Cor bovinum
- Brain decay
- Organ decay
- Fatty tissue contusions
- Inferior infarct
- Gunshot channel 1
- Gunshot channel 2
- SIDS overview
- Subdural hemorrhage

Conclusion

Modern radiological tomographic techniques, such as multi-slice CT and MRI, have yet to make inroads into daily routine work in clinical forensic medicine (examination of the living) or in classical forensic medicine (examination of the deceased). In the field of forensic virtual autopsy, imaging methods are currently used as supplementary examination tools or are evaluated as systematic postmortem examination methods in comparison with autopsy. It has to be assumed that multi-slice CT, thanks to its simpler operation, is set to supercede classical X-ray technology in forensic institutes.

As a result of the considerably higher costs and more demanding operation, MR technology will require a significantly longer time before it can be applied in postmortem routine diagnostics. An innovative and motivated radiology team for collaboration with forensic medicine is essential, as was realized in Berne.

An additional, but no less essential, problem of magnetic resonance imaging is that of examination times, which are still relatively long. However, with the recent introduction of spiral and moving-table MR technology, these times are being reduced to a level optimized to the procedure. The future potential of MR technology is very high, and it is not yet possible to assess its full potential from today's perspective. To cite just one example, with modern fiber-tracking methods it is possible to present lesions on the axon level [39].

Postmortem data can be gathered without being affected by the increasing trend to refuse autopsy (e.g. for religious reasons) in the population. Postmortem virtual autopsy can of course also be applied for highly infectious or chemically-biologically contaminated corpses (bioterrorism) with the concomitant advantages for the examiner. Imaging methods are suitable for forensic science, not least because data are collected without physical contact, non-invasively, and the stored data can be called up unchanged from the storage medium at any time for a second opinion or to facilitate a decisive expert opinion.

The knowledge verified by the correlation of radiology/pathology results has already had an impact on the interpretation of injury results from living victims of violence. The results form the basis for a scientific database of injury results that has been established in

Berne, which, in the future, will contribute to the training necessary in the new field of forensic radiology and the quality assurance in this discipline.

Thanks go to all Virtopsy research members/partners who have contributed to the project and to this article (cf. www.virtopsy.com), in particular to Dr. Christian Jackowski.

Bibliography

1. Brogdon BG. Forensic Radiology. 1st ed. Boca Raton, Florida, CRC Press LLC, 1998.
2. Farina J, Millana C, Fdez-Acenero MJ, Furio V, Aragoncillo P, Martin VG, Buencuerpo J. Ultrasonographic autopsy (echopsy): a new autopsy technique. Virchows Arch 2002; 440(6): 635–9.
3. Bratzke H, Schneider V, Dietz W. [Radiographic investigation during medico-legal autopsies (author's transl)]. Rofo 1982; 136(4): 463–72.
4. Clasen RA, Torack RM. Computerized tomography and neuropathologists: two viewpoints. J Neuropathol Exp Neurol 1982; 41(4): 387–8.
5. Schumacher M, Oehmichen M, Konig HG, Einighammer H. [Intravital and postmortem CT examinations in cerebral gunshot injuries]. ROFO Fortschr Geb Rontgenstr Nuklearmed 1983; 139(1): 58–62.
6. Schumacher M, Oehmichen M, Konig HG, Einighammer H, Bien S. [Computertomographic studies on wound ballistics of cranial gunshot injuries]. Beitr Gerichtl Med 1985; 43: 95–101.
7. Kalender WA, Seissler W, Klotz E, Vock P. Spiral volumetric CT with single-breath-hold technique, continuous transport, and continuous scanner rotation. Radiology 1990; 176(1): 181–3.
8. Ezawa H, Yoneyama R, Kandatsu S, Yoshikawa K, Tsujii H, Harigaya K. Introduction of autopsy imaging redefines the concept of autopsy: 37 cases of clinical experience. Pathol Int 2003; 53(12): 865–73.
9. Rutty GN, Swift B. Accuracy of magnetic resonance imaging in determining cause of sudden death in adults: comparison with conventional autopsy. Histopathology 2004; 44(2): 187–9.
10. Bisset RA, Thomas NB, Turnbull IW, Lee S. Postmortem examinations using magnetic resonance imaging: four year review of a working service. BMJ 2002; 324(7351): 1423–4.
11. Bisset RA. Magnetic resonance imaging may be alternative to necropsy. BMJ 1998; 317(7170): 1450.
12. Roberts IS, Benbow EW, Bisset R, Jenkins JP, Lee SH, Reid H, Jackson A. Accuracy of magnetic resonance imaging in determining cause of sudden death in adults: comparison with conventional autopsy. Histopathology 2003; 42(5): 424–30.
13. Patriquin L, Kassarjian A, Barish M, Casserley L, O'Brien M, Andry C, Eustace S. Postmortem whole-body magnetic resonance imaging as an adjunct to autopsy: preliminary clinical experience. J Magn Reson Imaging 2001; 13(2): 277–87.
14. Aghayev E, Yen K, Sonnenschein M, Ozdoba C, Thali M, Jackowski C, Dirnhofer R. Virtopsy post-mortem multi-slice computed tomography (MSCT) and magnetic resonance imaging (MRI) demonstrating descending tonsillar herniation: comparison to clinical studies. Neuroradiology 2004; 46(7): 559–64.
15. Jackowski C, Schweitzer W, Thali M, Yen K, Aghayev E, Sonnenschein M, Vock P, Dirnhofer R. Virtopsy: postmortem imaging of the human heart in situ using MSCT and MRI. Forensic Sci Int 2005; 149(1): 11–23.
16. Thali MJ, Yen K, Schweitzer W, Vock P, Boesch C, Ozdoba C, Schroth G, Ith M, Sonnenschein M, Doernhoefer T, Scheurer E, Plattner T, Dirnhofer R. Virtopsy, a new imaging horizon in forensic pathology: virtual autopsy by postmortem multislice computed tomography (MSCT) and magnetic resonance imaging (MRI) – a feasibility study. J Forensic Sci 2003; 48(2): 386–403.
17. Yen K, Vock P, Tiefenthaler B, Ranner G, Scheurer E, Thali MJ, Zwygart K, Sonnenschein M, Wiltgen M, Dirnhofer R. Virtopsy: forensic traumatology of the subcutaneous fatty tissue; multislice

computed tomography (MSCT) and magnetic resonance imaging (MRI) as diagnostic tools. J Forensic Sci 2004; 49(4): 799–806.

18. Yen K, Sonnenschein M, Thali MJ, Ozdoba C, Weis J, Zwygart K, Aghayev E, Jackowski C, Dirnhofer R. Postmortem Multislice Computed Tomography and Magnetic Resonance Imaging of odontoid fractures, atlantoaxial distractions and ascending medullary edema. Int J Legal Med 2005.

19. Amberg R, Forster B, Furmaier R. Identification by MRI. Z Rechtsmed 1989; 102(2–3): 185–9.

20. Ros PR, Li KC, Vo P, Baer H, Staab EV. Preautopsy magnetic resonance imaging: initial experience. Magn Reson Imaging 1990; 8(3): 303–8.

21. Brookes JA, Hall-Craggs MA, Sams VR, Lees WR. Non-invasive perinatal necropsy by magnetic resonance imaging. Lancet 1996; 348(9035): 1139–41.

22. Niermeijer MF. Perinatal necropsy by magnetic resonance imaging. Lancet 1997; 349(9044): 56.

23. Woodward PJ, Sohaey R, Harris DP, Jackson GM, Klatt EC, Alexander AL, Kennedy A. Postmortem fetal MR imaging: comparison with findings at autopsy. AJR Am J Roentgenol 1997; 168(1): 41–6.

24. Bruschweiler W, Braun M, Dirnhofer R, Thali MJ. Analysis of patterned injuries and injury-causing instruments with forensic 3D/CAD supported photogrammetry (FPHG): an instruction manual for the documentation process. Forensic Sci Int 2003; 132(2): 130–8.

25. Thali MJ, Braun M, Markwalder TH, Brueschweiler W, Zollinger U, Malik NJ, Yen K, Dirnhofer R. Bite mark documentation and analysis: the forensic 3D/CAD supported photogrammetry approach. Forensic Sci Int 2003; 135(2): 115–21.

26. Thali MJ, Braun M, Brueschweiler W, Dirnhofer R. "Morphological imprint": determination of the injury-causing weapon from the wound morphology using forensic 3D/CAD-supported photogrammetry. Forensic Sci Int 2003; 132(3): 177–81.

27. Thali MJ, Braun M, Bruschweiler W, Dirnhofer R. Matching tire tracks on the head using forensic photogrammetry. Forensic Sci Int 2000; 113(1–3): 281–7.

28. Thali MJ, Braun M, Dirnhofer R. Optical 3D surface digitizing in forensic medicine: 3D documentation of skin and bone injuries. Forensic Sci Int 2003; 137(2–3): 203–8.

29. Thali MJ, Braun M, Wirth J, Vock P, Dirnhofer R. 3D surface and body documentation in forensic medicine: 3-D/CAD Photogrammetry merged with 3D radiological scanning. J Forensic Sci 2003; 48(6): 1356–65.

30. Thali MJ, Yen K, Schweitzer W, Vock P, Ozdoba C, Dirnhofer R. Into the decomposed body-forensic digital autopsy using multislice-computed tomography. Forensic Sci Int 2003; 134(2–3): 109–14.

31. Thali MJ, Schweitzer W, Yen K, Vock P, Ozdoba C, Spielvogel E, Dirnhofer R. New horizons in forensic radiology: the 60-second digital autopsy-full-body examination of a gunshot victim by multislice computed tomography. Am J Forensic Med Pathol 2003; 24(1): 22–7.

32. Thali MJ, Yen K, Plattner T, Schweitzer W, Vock P, Ozdoba C, Dirnhofer R. Charred body: virtual autopsy with multi-slice computed tomography and magnetic resonance imaging. J Forensic Sci 2002; 47(6): 1326–31.

33. Thali M, Yen K, Vock P, Ozdoba C, Dirnhofer R. Image-guided virtual autopsy findings of gunshot victims performed with Multi-Slice Computed Tomography (MSCT) and Magnetic Resonance Imaging (MRI), and subsequent correlation between radiology and autopsy findings. Forensic Sci Int 2003.

34. Thali MJ, Taubenreuther U, Karolczak M, Braun M, Brueschweiler W, Kalender WA, Dirnhofer R. Forensic microradiology: micro-computed tomography (Micro-CT) and analysis of patterned injuries inside of bone. J Forensic Sci 2003; 48(6): 1336–42.

35. Thali MJ, Dirnhofer R, Becker R, Oliver W, Potter K. Is „virtual histology" the next step after the „virtual autopsy"? Magnetic resonance microscopy in forensic medicine. Magn Reson Imaging 2004; 22(8): 1131–8.

36. Jackowski C, Sonnenschein M, Thali M, Aghayev E, v. Almen G, Yen K, Dirnhofer R, Vock P. Virtopsy: Postmortem minimally invasive angiography using cross section techniques – implementation and preliminary results. J Forensic Med 2004; in print.

37. Aghayev E, Thali M, Jackowski C, Sonnenschein M, Yen K, Vock P, Dirnhofer R. Virtopsy – fatal motor vehicle accident with head injury. J Forensic Sci 2004; 49(4): 809–13.

38. Yen K, Thali M, Aghayev E, Jackowski C, Schweitzer W, Boesch C, Vock P, Dirnhofer R, Sonnenschein M. Strangulation signs – initial correlation of MRI/MSCT and forensic findings in nine deceased and two living patients. JMRI 2005; accepted.

39. Yen K, Kreis R, Weis J, Ozdoba C, Maier S, Dirnhofer R. DWI and DTI of the post-mortem brain: imaging, autopsy and histopathologic findings. Proc Intl Soc Magn Reson Med 2005; 13: 658.

Key word index

A

ADC image 19
Angio*SURF* XVIII, 29, 66, 133
ankylosing spondylitis 47, 58
Armes Forces Institute of Pathology
   (AFIP) 172
arterial hypertension 144
atherosclerosis 146, 153
–, peripheral 153
autopsy XIX

B

Baye's Theorem 146
Bechterew disease 58
bioelectric impedance analysis 114
blood sugar 88
body composition XIX
body mass index (BMI) 112
Body*SURF* 82
bone marrow 51
bone metastases XIX, 62, 65
bone scintigraphy 63, 65
BPH 132
brain infarct 177
BROCA 112

C

CAD 14
Cancer Screening Trial 139
carcinoma
–, bone metastases 51
–, breast 51, 130, 146, 151
–, bronchial 51, 73, 129, 146, 151
–, cervical 147
–, colon 146, 152
–, colorectal 130
–, larynx 105

–, prostate 51, 105, 131, 151
–, thyroid 51
–, renal 51
cardiovascular diseases 33
cerebrovascular diseases 154
32-channel MR systems 89
chronic lymphocytic leukemia 108
claudication 44
client 145
coil
–, matrix 7
–, surface 5
–, peripheral 6
–, phased-array 5
–, RF transmit 12
colonoscopy 102
computed tomography (CT) XVII
connective tissue disease 57
contrast agents XVII
conventional colonography 152
cor bovinum 176
coronary arteries 34
coronary heart disease 28, 112, 153
costs 146

D

DEXA (dual-energy X-ray absorptiometry) 112, 114
densitometry 113
dermatitis 59
diabetes 44
–, mellitus 145
DICOM 21f
digital subtraction angiography (DSA) 28f
distortion correction 4
dyslipidemia 112